Sociocultural Implications in Treatment Planning in Occupational Therapy

The *Occupational Therapy in Health Care* series,
Florence S. Cromwell, Editor

Sociocultural Implications in Treatment Planning in Occupational Therapy

Florence S. Cromwell
Editor

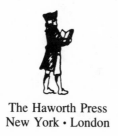

The Haworth Press
New York • London

Sociocultural Implications in Treatment Planning in Occupational Therapy has also been published as *Occupational Therapy in Health Care,* Volume 4, Number 1, Spring 1987.

The Haworth Press, Inc., 12 West 32 Street, New York, NY 10001
EUROSPAN/Haworth, 3 Henrietta Street, London WC2E 8LU England

Library of Congress Cataloging-in-Publication Data

Sociocultural implications in planning treatment in occupational therapy.

   "Has also been published as Occupational therapy in health care, volume 4, number 1, spring 1987"—T.p. verso.
   Includes bibliographies.
   1. Occupational therapy—Planning—Social aspects. 2. Minorities—Medical care.
I. Cromwell, Florence S.
[DNLM: 1. Occupational Therapy. 2. Patient Care Planning—methods.
3. Socioeconomic Factors.
W1 OC601H v.4 no. 1 / WB 555 S678]
RM735.S57   1987   615.8'5152   86-31827
ISBN 0-86656-612-0

Sociocultural Implications in Treatment Planning in Occupational Therapy

Occupational Therapy in Health Care
Volume 4, Number 1

CONTENTS

PRACTICE WATCH: THINGS TO THINK ABOUT

BOOK REVIEWS

Sociocultural Implications in Treatment Planning in Occupational Therapy

FROM THE EDITOR'S DESK

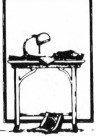

Volume IV starts on a high note bringing to readers in this first issue timely information on a topic that strikes at the core of occupational therapy practice. Our beliefs as occupational therapists in holism and our professed concern for addressing the needs of the person in *his* own own setting can only be exercised if we attend to the sociocultural aspects of our patients' makeup. Thus this issue is devoted to helping readers achieve a richer knowledge and understanding about culture, its influences, and of the broad fabric which many of us find in our caseloads today.

With the theme thoughtfully introduced by Levine, the issue moves to papers which address many, though not certainly all, of the major cultures we need to know about today: Hispanic/Latino, Asian (Japanese, Chinese, Filipino, Southeast Asian), Black, Appalachian, Native Canadian, and indeed the "usual" American patient who has his own unique values and lifestyle. Specific health beliefs and practices of different cultures are discussed in many papers.

Skawski reminds us, however, with the report of her study, that we as occupational therapists have not been as attentive to our patients' values as we might in planning their treatment programs. Gill provides a new dimension to our thinking about the culture of the disabled in a thought-provoking piece on social perspectives on disability.

Papers are both informative and with very practical content as programs are described, or cases discussed. I believe you will find the reading interesting and useful. Our *Practice Watch* feature presents a stimulating paper on Wellness and about the relationship of occupational therapy to this emerging interest among those of all ages. The issue concludes with some book reviews on a diverse set of titles.

Looking ahead to the rest of Volume IV brings promise of three other issues on very popular areas of interest among occupational therapists with titles of: *Sensory Integrative Approaches in Occupational Therapy, The Occupational Therapy Manager's Survival Handbook* and *Hand Rehabilitation in Occupational Therapy.* Watch for them.

Florence S. Cromwell
Editor

Culture: A Factor Influencing the Outcomes of Occupational Therapy

Ruth E. Levine, EdD, OTR/L, FAOTA

ABSTRACT. Culture is defined and discussed as an important ingredient to treatment planning. Components of culture are identified and examples of how they pertain to treatment are given through a brief case example.

OVERVIEW

People can accomplish seemingly impossible goals if invested in the outcome; on the other hand, few people are interested in activities that have no personal meaning. This paper will explore one of the factors that can make therapy more meaningful to our patients. The concept is a complex pattern of living which is called culture. As therapists, we search for activities that will stimulate and interest our patients as well as promote functional abilities. This is no easy task because few of our patients come from the same culture group that we do. This paper will define culture, review the importance of culture in occupational therapy practice, and describe how cultural beliefs and values affect assessment and treatment in occupational therapy.

Let us begin with a treatment vignette that offers an introduction to the concept of culture.

Case Study. Mrs. W., a 57 year old, attractive, upper-middle class, urban housewife, suffered from Guillian-Barre syndrome,

Ruth E. Levine is Professor and Chairman, Department of Occupational Therapy, College of Allied Health Sciences, Thomas Jefferson University, Philadelphia, PA.

This article appears jointly in *Sociocultural Implications in Treatment Planning in Occupational Therapy* (The Haworth Press, Inc., 1987) and in *Occupational Therapy in Health Care*, Volume 4, Number 1 (Spring 1987).

3

was hospitalized and transferred to a rehabilitation center and then to home care. Mrs. W. occupied a first-floor bedroom suite in the newly purchased home of one of her daughters. The family reasoned that Mrs. W. could interact with family members, walk short distances and join the family for meals. The physical therapist felt that Mrs. W. was almost ready to return to her own home if it were adapted to accommodate Mrs. W.'s needs. Mrs. W. lived in a newly constructed three story townhouse in center city. Although the OTR felt that referral to occupational therapy was perhaps too late for best results, she decided to visit the patient anyway.

On the day of the scheduled evaluation visit, the OTR was admitted into the gracious house by the maid because the daughter was conferring with an interior decorator. The OTR was led to the first floor bedroom where Mrs. W. was propped up in bed while a full time attendant fussed over her sheets and cleared her breakfast dishes. Mrs. W. ignored the therapist and continued her conversation with the attendant. After a few minutes, Mrs. W. briefly acknowledged the OTR and spent the next fifteen minutes describing her symptoms as if the OTR was an unwanted, inexperienced newcomer. Mrs. W. praised "her" physical therapist and attributed her progress to his guidance and skill. The occupational therapist tried to guide their conversation toward the patient's previous interests and activities and her present views on self-care and independence, but Mrs. W. switched the conversation back to the physical therapist.

The OTR decided to define her role and the type of equipment that might improve Mrs. W.'s functional abilities. This seemed to make Mrs. W. act more defensively. The OTR tried to ameliorate her discomfort by pointing out useful safety rails and tub seats in an equipment catalog. Mrs. W. grew even more negative and told the OTR that she did not need adaptive equipment. The OTR soon realized that something was wrong with the interview but could not fathom why it was going so poorly. Mrs. W. became more upset as the therapist tried to win her approval by switching the topic to the other services offered by an occupational therapist including work simplification and analysis of architectural barriers. Unfortunately, this topic also proved difficult and Mrs. W. interrupted the OTR and told her that the physical therapist said that she was making excellent progress. The OTR tried to explain that she was impressed with Mrs. W.'s efforts but this praise did not impress Mrs. W.

The OTR decided there was nothing else to do so she concluded the evaluation by telling Mrs. W. that she would close the case since Mrs. W. had no interest in adaptive equipment. Mrs. W. said she hoped that she would never see the occupational therapist again and told the OTR that she planned to report her to the physical therapist. Later, the physical therapist called the OTR to find out what had gone wrong with the evaluation. He reported that Mrs. W. was angry and upset and claimed that the OTR insisted that she would need "handicapped" equipment for the rest of her life. The OTR was both hurt and confused and wondered what she had done to infuriate Mrs. W. After all, she was doing exactly what she had been taught in her training for home health care.

The negative outcome of this evaluation visit affected all of the team members—patient, caretakers, physical therapist, nurse and the occupational therapist. Each person was interpreting events from their own perspective. The meaning of the communication was, in part, determined by the person's values, interests, goals, roles and habits. Each person's culture became a filter or screen that either passed information through or blocked it. The vignette demonstrates that even though the therapist's professional manner was similar to that prescribed during her professional training, the patient interpreted the visit as an attempt to jinx her hard won progress. In retrospect, the OTR may have realized that two different opinions about the value of adaptive equipment started the tangled communication. Within a short time, the OTR could not extricate herself from the negative meaning that "handicapped" things had for Mrs. W. The therapist moved her treatment agenda too quickly without hearing what the patient was really saying. Mrs. W. was frightened by her diagnosis and did not want to see, touch, own, or talk about anything that implied that she might not regain her independence. In Mrs. W.'s culture outward appearances were of vital importance, people who used adaptive equipment were handicapped and the thought that other people might regard her as disabled was more stressful than being dependent on an attendant.

HISTORICAL OVERVIEW

Occupational therapy founders first considered culture as an important aspect of treatment planning because of their belief in the interrelationship between mind and body. If an activity generated a patient's interests it could also promote functional independence. In the first occupations training course, Tracy identified activities that matched the patient's lifestyle[1] and Dunton agreed and emphasized the need to stimulate the patient's interests by prescribing activities based on personal and cultural values.[2] Hall and Buck claimed that "brain workers should be given work that was largely physical and those who worked with their hands, must have simpler, more primitive tasks."[3] Although the consideration of culture was not fully developed, the Founders searched for different ways to elicit a patient's interest through the use of novel experiences. In 1925 a committee of the American Occupational Therapy Association defined occupational therapy and formulated fifteen principles of which one-third emphasized the importance of considering the patient's interests and needs.[4] Thus, the early literature of the profession is filled with examples of attempts to consider the patient's culture during treatment.

As medical care became more scientific in the 1930's and 1940's, therapists began to concentrate more on the patient's pathology than on residual strengths; thus, decreasing their initial commitment to linking the patient's goals, interests and values, habits and roles with the activity process. At the same time, many therapists were arts-and-crafts teachers who were committed to a philosophy that tended to encourage patients to refine their craft skills and produce an attractive end-product. It was believed that the quality product would enhance self-confidence. Other therapists concentrated on the benefits that occurred during the *doing* part of the activity process. Thus, ideological differences grew between the therapists and the diversionists.[5] Another factor that compromised initial consideration of culture during the Depression years was the scarcity of funds. Therapists had to treat large numbers of patients and market and sell patient projects in order to replenish department supply budgets. The patients' interests were subordinated to the department needs since some projects were more cost efficient than others.

The emphasis on arts-and-crafts with little concentration on the therapeutic use of activities may have prompted Eleanor Clarke Slagle to tell the 1930 graduating class at Sheppard and Enoch Pratt Hospital that "handicrafts are not enough" because " . . . the patient is being more and more considered in relation to his domestic and community life."[6]

Culture was as important in early practice as it must be today, because occupational therapy deals with goal-directed activities which are part and parcel of everyday life. Recently, modern therapists are rediscovering the importance of early beliefs that emphasized the interaction of mind and body during treatment. Theorists Mosey,[7] Fidler,[8] Llorens,[9] Reilly,[10] Keilhofner and Burke,[11,12] Barris,[13] Nuse-Clark,[14] and Yerxa,[15] all address the influence of culture in treatment. Using basic concepts from our past, present-day theorists still emphasize the importance of the patient's motivation, interests, goals, interests, values, habits, time-orientation, roles, caretaker network and use of the non-human environment. All of these concepts are part of a person's culture.

DEFINING CULTURE

Culture has been described as a "blueprint" for human behavior, influencing individual thoughts, actions and collectively influencing a particular society.[16] Culture can be viewed as a multifaceted influence which is learned by direct and indirect daily experiences based on what people do (cultural behavior), say (speech messages), make and use (cultural artifacts). In short, a child learns a life pattern of beliefs and values which shape the way that he or she believes, thinks, perceives, feels and behaves.[17] Culture is a way of life which encompasses kinetic or overt behavior, psychological expressions and the material products of labor or industry. The major cultural transmission agents are behavioral and material elements simply because psychological states are not transferable.[18]

Kinetic or overt behaviors, the first elements of culture, are evident in actions performed by an individual and include: body motions, speech patterns, distance selected during communication with others and use of products and tools. People use their bodies in unique ways to indicate agreement, acceptance, rejection, discomfort and other reactions.

Speech patterns are also culturally determined; rate of speech, expression and emphasis, pronunciation, and choice of words are part of a person's culture. Even the distance preferred between people during different activities is also culturally determined.[19] Tool use, as part of one's behavior, is another factor indigenous to one's culture: some people use handtools exclusively, others rely on sophisticated gadgets and technology, some others prefer to use only their hands in doing tasks. In examining culture one must also consider how people employ objects and other artifacts. For example, consider a patient who uses the same hammer over and over and seems to derive pleasure from completing a task by using this object which almost seems like a non-human friend. In contrast, another patient may be careless with tools and abuse them without giving it a second thought. Still another patient may regard the use of tools with disdain since handmade objects can be purchased and "time is money."

Psychological aspects, the second elements of one's culture, include knowledge, attitudes and values that are shared by members of a given cultural group. These factors cannot be readily observed since they take place in a person's mind. Psychological factors are therefore more difficult for an observer to assess and observe. Although these factors are subjective they still deserve some of our attention since people exibit different reactions to events in their daily lives. On the other hand, measurement of psychological factors is not precise and individual reactions may be inconsistent and variable even under the same circumstances. For example, if you introduce yourself to a patient using your first name only some people may feel right at home, welcome your informality and respond with warmth and humor. On the other hand, another person may find it annoying but tolerable and respond stiffly to requests for additional information. We can speculate that the first patient equates the informality with a type of relationship where the therapist and he are equal partners. The second patient may feel that she has just met the therapist and the use of first names indicates a forced familiarity that makes the patient feel guarded. Thus we see that the same event can take on different meaning for each participant depending on one's cultural background.

The last element associated with culture, the "material products of labor or industry," are the objects and artifacts that comprise *the non-human environment.* This category includes signs, symbols, objects, tasks, roles and social organizations used to create products in the environment. Consider the work produced by a given group of people, the way that ideas are transformed into reality and the type of organization that is needed to produce the goods and services. Members of a group teach their children how to participate in their culture through a complex system of rewards and punishments which are conveyed through thoughts, actions, social beliefs, attitudes, communication patterns, perceptions, time orientation and ways of handling animals, plants and objects. In effect, a child is exposed to a pattern of beliefs, attitudes, perceptions, meanings and emotions based on personal experiences in a particular setting.[20]

Culture imposes a conditioning variable that is internalized in the human psyche and not easily forgotten.[21] Values, interests, goals, habits, roles, time orientation, communication patterns, the ways in which one uses symbols and artifacts, selects non-human objects— all are well ingrained as one grows, making change difficult. In fact, Likroeber compared culture to the great coral reefs built by polyps. The polyps die but their secretions leave a permanent record of their former life.[22] Thus, culture establishes a filter through which individuals interpret daily events. At the same time, one's group establishes patterns that become "commonly defined meanings and sanctioned behaviors favored by the group."[23] Individual are never free of the group influence—sometimes subtle and sometimes more specialized—to meet individual physical and psychological needs.[24]

THE RELEVANCE OF CULTURE
IN OCCUPATIONAL THERAPY

Culture is a central component of occupational therapy because people judge the quality of their therapy through a filter which is comprised, in part, of past learning and emotions and which is based on three levels of beliefs: (1) the patient's perception of illness and health, (2) the patient's perception of therapy, and (3) the patient's belief in the meaning of his own life and activities. These factors overlap and are not discrete.

Illness is not the same to all individuals. Sociologists have long identified significant differences in the ways that members of specific cultures decide to: seek health care, care for themselves, use family caretaker networks, take medication and follow pre- scribed remedies, participate in a healthful daily regime, assist other ill family members and endure pain and suffering.[25,26,27,28,29,30] Occupational therapists can not assume that people all react to the stress of illness, traumatic events or other life disruptions in the same way. "Illness behavior" refers to the ways in which symp- toms may be differently perceived, evaluated and acted (or not acted) upon by different kinds of persons.[31] The behavior varies with a person's socioeconomic class, education level, community cohesiveness and ethnic origin. The higher the social status of a population, the better educated and informed they will be about signs and symptoms of illness.[32]

Being "ill" certainly is not the same to everyone. Some people are not ill until they are incapable of performing daily roles, others are ill as soon as they note a slight change in their body, still others are ill only if the illness is labeled by the medical establishment and therefore given "official" sanction. Therapists must consider the issue of illness behavior in rehabiliation because of diverse reactions such as a patient who does not want to participate in therapy because he is "ill" and therefore is not *capable* of participation. This type of behavior was described in a case study depicting the progress of an elderly Italian-American, with a left hemiparesis, who maintained that he could not dress or toilet himself until his arm "got well." This response is logical if you understand the culture of the first-generation, Southern Italian.[33,34]

Another question to consider is how well patients understand their treatment programs. Occupational therapy can only be perceived as meaningful, and deserving of the patient's interest and cooperation if it is relevant to patients and their caretakers. Treatment is valued only if patients believe that they have been helped by it. If not, services are judged as irrelevant and inconsequential. Chances are that therapists who are capable of attending to the patient's cultural values by selecting relevant treatment activities are also able to convince the patient that therapy is important. Yet, it is difficult to tap into the interests of patients who have experienced a traumatic illness, accident or event which has drained their energies and made adaptation seem overwhelming and taxing. Sharrott maintained that occupational therapists "play a profound role in creation, affirmation and experience of meaning" since therapy provides opportunities for patients to redefine their previous experiences in light of their present abilities and needs.[35] Effective therapy alters the patient's perception of meaningful existence by offering concrete feedback on daily performance in activities that are important in a patient's life roles. Unlike other treatment, occupational therapy mirrors the painful limitations wrought by tramatic incident, aging, development or deprivation. But therapy sessions can alter the patient's perception of life by providing immediate evidence on what the patient *CAN* do rather than what is lost.[36]

Another factor, frequently overlooked when designing therapy programs is the patient's beliefs and values regarding the nonhuman environment. Barris discussed the importance of the treatment environment because it should provide "adequate but not overbearing stimulation."[37] Patients will express culturally determined values about their environment and these ideas should be respected. For example, some patients prefer to do their therapy activities alone and refuse to participate in a group project whereas other patients like to be involved in the social interactions that evolve during work on a collective project. Relevance or the link between therapy and the patient's reality, should become part of initial treatment planning because the therapist is responsible for developing a strong link between the patient's interests and the goals of the occupational therapy program. This is not to say that it is easy to develop therapy that is compatible with the patient's goals, values and interests. These three factors: the patient's perception of illness and health, the patient's perception of therapy and the patient's belief in the meaning of life and activities are all considered in a successful therapy program.

FACTORS TO CONSIDER DURING EVALUATION AND TREATMENT

This section will use information presented in the earlier case study to demonstrate how the OTR could have improved her assessment if cultural factors had been considered during the evaluation visit.

Conceptual Framework. One way to systematically include culture in one's daily treatment is to select a conceptual framework or model that includes culture. Although many occupational therapy theories and models mention culture, the Model of Human Occupation[38,39] includes a conceptual structure that integrates data about the patient's values, goals, interests, personal causation, habits and roles into occupational therapy.

Background. The next step is to observe and investigate the lifestyle of cultural group members. Consider the largest number of ethnic group members in your patient load and find out where group members live. Try to do a small-scale, informal ethnographic study by exploring a local store, restaurant, recreational center or religious sanctuary.[40] During your visit use your clinical skills to observe the human and non-human environment and the way that group members interact. Consider the values that are conveyed through all of these cues.

For instance, if the OTR had visited Mrs. W.'s neighborhood, she would have found a row of exclusive townhouses in a village within center city. The colonial-style, three-story, brick houses have narrow stairways and small rooms—in no way a barrier-free environment. Each house faced an attractive courtyard with a few trees and benches in the center. Garages were hidden underground and could only be accessed by an enclosed walkway. The houses were situated near a cluster of exclusive stores where one could buy things like gourmet take-out food, imported wine, custom made tiles, designer clothing or hand-made lampshades.

This uppermiddle-class neighborhood conveyed an air of cosmopolitan homogeneity. Although the OTR could not assume that Mrs. W. shared all of her neighbors' values, she could still learn something about her patient's lifestyle. It is not realistic to visit every patient's neighborhood; nonetheless, one can choose the largest group among one's patients and gather some background information about them. This data is as important as looking up medication side-effects and unfamiliar medical diagnoses.

Reading offers another source of information. Research on particular cultural groups appears in sociological, anthropological and historical journals. Books also depict life in a particular culture. For instance, Chute's novel about the pain, humiliation and rage of a poverty-stricken New England family[41] offers insight into rural deprivation. Factual accounts are also useful, such as the story told by Wideman, a Black-American Rhodes scholar and English professor, who searches for an answer to why his brother who was raised by the same parents in the same environment as the author is presently serving a life sentence for murder.[42] Television and film documentaries that portray family and community life are helpful in understanding different lifestyles. In short, the OTR should gather as much information as possible about a patient's cultural group before the evaluation visit.

Using the case-study as an example, the OTR did not adequately prepare for the evaluation visit. The nurse and the physical therapist could have been used as informants so the OTR could be introduced to the patient's lifestyle. The OTR tried to control the interview by taking charge and asking questions. Mrs. W. valued competition and outward appearances; moreover, it was important for her to act like the family matriarch. Thus, the OTR became a rival. During the first fifteen minutes of the interview, the OTR could have satisfied Mrs. W.'s need for attention by listening to her description of her progress and offering support for her efforts. At the same time, the OTR could have throughly observed the environment.

Evaluation. The initial evaluation is a crucial time to establish trust and gather cues from the human and the non-human environment. There are a number of evaluation tools that can be used to direct these observations. Use a guide to begin your search for an effective instrument. The Kielhofner text *The Model of Human Occupation*[43] includes an overview of assessment tools or Asher's *Annotated Index of Occupational Therapy Evaluation Tools*[44] which includes profiles on 87 occupational therapy instruments, as well as information on where to find the tool.

Since no instrument is perfect, consider elements of the patient's lifestyle by observing values concerning life, death, health, productivity, work, family relations, human nature, time, meaningful activities and religion. Be alert to ethnic myths and taboos which will impede care if misunderstood by the therapist. Use data gathered from the evaluation tools you use to refine your ideas about treatment. For example, Mrs. W. may have responded better if the OTR had explored one of her interests and then used the activity to observe Mrs. W.'s functional abilities.

Specific tools which could have been used in conjunction with other ADL, cognitive, perceptual or motor evaluations are the Occupational Role History,[45,46] a semi-structured interview on occupational choice, work experience and leisure satisfaction, or The Occupational Questionnaire[47] which collects data on the patient's use of time in daily activities and how that relates to the patient's values, interests and personal causation. Two other useful tools are The Role Checklist which assesses productive adult life-roles by indicating the individual's perceptions of past, present, and future roles[48] and the Time Battery for gathering qualitative and quantitative data on temporal adaptation and use of time.[49] The OTR should have selected a tool which seemed to provide appropriate ideas for treatment planning.

Even if the OTR had used better interviewing skills, completed an ADL Evaluation and administered an instrument such as the Occupational Questionnaire, she would still need to compare this data with cues from the environment. Thus, the OTR's observation skills are fundamental to evaluation and treatment planning because patients may not always mean what they say. Examine the "extent to which the patient's beliefs, values, and customs are congruent with a trifold set of standards: from the patient's culture or ethnic group, from the therapist's own culture, and from the setting in which the treatment takes place."[50] Consider the extent that the patient is "like all other humans, like some other humans, and like no other humans."[51] Take time to identify and label similarities and differences between the patient's culture and the therapist's. This will help to separate personal bias and needs from those of the patient. For example, not all patients want to be independent in self-care. Some want to direct their energies toward other activities and view assistance as a trade-off. This was certainly true for Mrs. W.

A final consideration is the setting in which treatment takes place. Is the therapist a guest in the patient's home or is the patient a visitor in the hospital? The answer to those questions will determine roles and relationships. Treatment must be appropriate for the setting. For example, the institution is not always the best place to teach cooking and toileting skills since the information must be retaught once the patient returns home. On the other hand, the home setting is not suitable for constructing complex equipment and hand splints.

SUMMARY

This paper has explored the importance of culture in occupational therapy. Occupational therapy founders emphasized the need to consider the patient's interests in treatment. Today, we again realize that treatment must be meaningful to patients. Thus, cultural factors must be considered in evaluation and treatment. This is no easy task since we are all entrenched in our own value systems. However, although there are many differences among cultural groups there are also many similarities. Occupations can serve as a "common light among cultures."[52]

N.B. Throughout this paper the author has used the term "patient" to refer to the recipient of treatment. The term client was eschewed because it did not reflect people who were receiving medical services.

REFERENCES

1. Tracy, SE: *Studies in invalid occupations.* Boston: Whitcomb and Barrows. 1912

2. Dunton, WR: *Occupational Therapy: A manual for nurses.* Philadelphia: WB Saunders Co. 1918

3. Hall, H and Buck, MMC: *Handicrafts for the Handicapped.* New York: Moffatt, Yard and Company, 1916, p. xii

4. American Occupational Therapy Association Committee. An outline of lectures in Occupational Therapy to medical students and physicians. *Occupational Therapy and Rehabilitation. 5,* 1925, p. 278

5. Doane, JC: Presidential address delivered at AOTA annual meeting, Toronto, Canada, September 28–30, 1931. Reprinted in *Occupational Therapy and Rehabiliation 10* 1931, p. 365

6. Slagle, EC: Address to Graduates, Sheppard and Enoch Pratt Hospital, Towson, Maryland. June 28, 1930. *Occupational Therapy and Rehabilitation. 9* 1930, p. 275

7. Mosey, AC: *Occupational Therapy: Configuration of a Profession.* New York: Raven Press, 1981. p. 78

8. Fidler, GS and Fidler, JW: Doing and becoming: the Occupational Therapy experience. In Kielhofner, G, *Health through occupation.* Philadelphia: FA Davis Company, 1983, p. 267–280

9. Llorens, LA: *Application of a developmental theory for health and rehabilitation.* American Occupational Therapy Association. 1976

10. Reilly, M: The modernization of Occupational Therapy. *Amer J Occup Ther 25,* 1971, p. 243–246

11. Keilhofner, G and Burke, JP: Components and determinants of human occupation. In Kielhofner, G (Editor): *A model of human occupation: theory and application.* Baltimore, Maryland: Williams and Wilkins. 1985, p. 12–36

12. Kielhofner, G and Burke, JP: A model of human occupation, Part 1. Conceptual Framework and content. *Amer J Occup Ther 34,* 1980, pp. 572–581

13. Barris, R: Environmental interactions: an extension of the model of occupation. *Amer J Occup Ther 36,* 1982, pp

14. Nuse-Clark, P: Human development through occupation: A philosophy and conceptual model for practice, part 2. *Amer J Occup Ther 33,* 1979, pp. 577–585

15. Yerxa, E: Audicious values: the energy source for occupational therapy practice. In Kielhofner, G. (Editor) *Health through occupation.* Philadelphia: FA Davis, 1983. pp. 149–162

16. Leininger, M: *Transcultural nursing: concepts, theories and practices.* New York: John Wiley and Sons. 1978, p. 80

17. Spradley, JP, McDurdy, DW (Editors): *Conformity and conflict.* Boston: Little, Brown, 1980, p. 2

18. Linton, R. *The cultural background of personality.* New York: Appleton-Century-Crofts, Inc. 1945, p. 38

19. Hall, ET: *The hidden dimension.* Garden City, New York: Anchor Books, 1969

20. Laudin, H: *Victims of culture.* Columbus, Ohio: Charles E. Merrill Pub. co. 1973

21. Opler, M: *Culture and social psychiatry.* New York: Atherton Press. 1967, p. 14

22. Likroeber, AI: quoted in Laudin, op. cit. p. 4

23. Ibid, p. 184

24. Ibid, p. 189

25. Mechanic, D: Response factors in illness: the study of illness behavior. in Jaco, EG, (Editor): *Patients, physicians and illness.* New York: The Free Press. 1972, pp. 128–141

26. Leininger, op. cit.

27. Saunders, L: *Cultural difference and medical care.* New York: Russell Sage Foundation. 1954

28. Scott, CS: Health and healing practices among five ethnic groups in Miami, Florida. *Public Health Reports.* 89 1974, pp. 524–32

29. Suchman, EA: Social patterns of illness and medical care. *Journal of health and human behavior. 6,* 1965, pp. 2–16

30. Wolff, BB and Langley, S: Cultural factors and the response to pain. A review. In Weisenberg, M (Editor): *Pain: clinical and experimental perspectives.* Saint Louis: The CV Mosby Co. 1975, pp. 141–143

31. Mechanic, D. Religion, religiousity, and illness behavior. *Human organization. 22,* 1963, p. 202

32. Suchman, EA: Sociomedical variations among ethic groups. *American Journal of Sociology. 70* 1964–5, pp. 319–331

33. Lopreato, J: *Italian Americans.* New York: Random House, 1970

34. Levine, RE: The cultural aspects of home care delivery. *Amer J Occup Ther 38,* 1984, pp. 736–737

35. Sharrott, G: Occupational therapy's role in the client's creation and affirmation of meaning. In Kielhofner, G: *Health through occupation.* Philadelphia: FA Davis. 1983, p. 215

36. Rogers, JC: The spirit of independence: the evolution of a philosophy. *Amer J Occup Ther 36,* 1982 pp. 709–715

37. Barris, op. cit.

38. Kielhofner and Burke, op. cit.

39. Kielhofner, G, op. cit.

40. Merrill, SC: Qualitative methods in occupational therapy research: an application. *The occupational therapy journal of research.* 5 1985, pp. 209–222

41. Chute, C: *The Beans of Egypt, Maine.* New York: Ticknor & Fields, 1985

42. Wideman, JE: *Brothers and keepers.* New York: Penguin Books, 1984

43. Kielhofner, op. cit.

44. Asher, IE: *Annotated index of Occupational Therapy evaluation tools.* Thomas Jefferson University, Department of Occupational Therapy, 1985

45. Moorehead, L: The occupational history. *Amer J Occup Ther 23,* 1969, pp. 329–334

46. Florey, LL & Michelman, SM: Occupational role history: a screening tool for psychiatric occupational therapy. *Amer J Occup Ther 36,* 1982 pp. 301–8

47. Riopel, N & Kielhofner, G: Occupational questionnaire. In Asher, op. cit. p. 57

48. Oakley, F: The role checklist. In Asher, op. cit. p. 58

49. Larrington, G: Time Battery. In Asher, op. cit. p. 59

50. Tripp-Reimer, T., Brink, PJ, Saunders, JM: Cultural assessment: content and process. *Nursing Outlook. 32,* p. 81

51. Kluckholn, C: quoted in Brill, NI: *Working with people: the helping process.* Philadelphia: JB Lippincott, 1976, p. 19

52. Malinowski, B: *Argonauts of the western pacific.* New York: EP Dutton and Co., Inc., 1961, p. 25

Culture and Communication in the Treatment Planning for Occupational Therapy With Minority Patients

Guy L. McCormack, MS, OTR

ABSTRACT. Ethnic minority populations are increasing in health care delivery systems. Statistics show that ethnic minorities have a greater need for health care but have not received comparable services as those afforded to the white middle class majority. This paper provides information on the characteristics, health beliefs and practices of Hispanic, Indochinese, Asians (Japanese, Chinese and Filipinos) and Black Americans. Effective treatment planning is contingent upon the recognition of these beliefs and cultural values. Strategies for intercultural communication as a guide to promoting better occupational therapy services to ethnic minorities will be provided.

In recent years, there has been a dramatic increase of ethnic minority populations in the health care system. Statistics indicate that health care needs of ethnic minorities are far greater than those of the dominant white majority in the United States. Ethnic minorities have a higher incidence of maternal mortality, cerebrovascular and cardiovascular disease and malignant neoplasms. Their life span is 4.9 to 5.8 years shorter than that of the white population.[1]

In 1980, the U.S. Public Health Service published an important report entitled "Promoting Health/Preventing Disease".[2] This lengthy document was based on findings in the 1970's which

---

Guy L. McCormack is Assistant Professor, San Jose State University, Department of Occupational Therapy, San Jose, CA.

This article appears jointly in *Sociocultural Implications in Treatment Planning in Occupational Therapy* (The Haworth Press, Inc., 1987) and in *Occupational Therapy in Health Care* Volume 4, Number 1 (Spring 1987)

17

indicated that the knowledge of health promotion and disease prevention could further reduce unnecessary death and disability in the United States. The objectives and the implementation plans described in this document represent early steps to improved health status in America. Unfortunately, despite the widely accepted belief that health care is the right of all Americans, the health status of ethnic minorities suggests that they are far from achieving this right.

Available statistics indicate that this problem may get worse because of increased immigration patterns and the influx of illegal aliens. The provisional 1980 census count shows the fastest growing minority group in the United States are Hispanic (Latino) Americans.[3] This is a culturally diverse group accounting for 14.6 million individuals. Needless to say, this count is far from accurate because it does not include those who have migrated to the United States without obtaining citizenship. Hispanic Americans include persons who have migrated from Mexico, Cuba, Puerto Rico, the Caribbean, South and Central America.[4]

Another large population are the Southeast (Indochinese) Asian refugees. Since 1975, 631,544 Indochinese Asians have resettled in the United States. This group is composed primarily of Vietnamese, Cambodians, Hmong and Laotians. Most of these refugees from Indochina have settled in the Western part of the United States; one third reside in California.[5]

The "established" Asian Americans are composed of Japanese, Chinese, Filipinos and Pacific Islanders. Collectively, this group constitutes approximately 1,909,027 citizens in the United States.[6] Black Americans represent 26,488,218 or 11.7% of the population of the United States. Approximately 53% of the 26 million Black American continue to live in the Southeastern region of the United States.[7]

Based on the available statistics and demographic information, the so-called ethnic minority populations are growing. This suggests that health care should be delivered in terms that recognize their beliefs and cultural values. Each ethnic minority group has unique health care needs. Health professionals should heighten their knowledge of different cultural groups and enhance their ability to communicate to members of other cultures.

The purpose of the paper is twofold. First, the paper will provide background information on the characteristics, health beliefs and practices of selected ethnic minority groups most likely to be treated by occupational therapists. Second, the paper will provide basic principles and techniques in intercultural communication to augment successful interpersonal relationships for treatment planning.

MULTICULTURAL HEALTH BELIEFS AND PRACTICES—CULTURAL DIVERSITY

Occupational therapists in the United States are working in a culturally diverse society. Therapists are more likely to have contact with patients of ethnic minorities than ever before. In order to meet the total needs of their clients/patients, occupational therapists will have to become sensitive to different cultural values, beliefs and practices. It will also be important to avoid generalizations which, in fact, may not apply universally to all groups. As we try to categorize groups into Hispanic, Indochinese, Blacks and established Asians, we run the risk of stereotyping. Ruhly[8] defines stereotypes as beliefs about groups of individuals or objects. Therefore, stereotypes are based on previously formed opinions or habits of perceiving. In some ways, stereotyping satisfies the human need to organize the unknown. In order to understand an ethnic group we may have to identify them in terms of their most basic or widely believed characteristics. For example Blacks are good athletes, Mexicans are modest and Asians are quiet. These are hasty generalizations that can lead to oversimplification of a person or ethnic group and deny the opportunity to learn about the uniqueness of each individual. The therapist should look beyond the information that supports a stereotype of an ethnic group and realize that there are individual variations within each ethnic group.

Ethnocentrism is another attitude to avoid. This a deeply ingrained belief that one's own culture is superior to another. According to Porter,[9] ethnocentrism is the tendency to judge people, their environments and their communication according to the standards, customs, and values of one's own culture. In the United States the standard is often based on the values of the white middle class majority. This attitude predisposes minority groups who are different, "culturally deprived" or "inferior". Therefore it is important for occupational therapists to keep an open mind by withholding judgments until more information is obtained on belief systems of minority patients.

Prejudice is another barrier to communication which stems from stereotyped beliefs, but tends to be more of an attitude. Prejudice has been defined as a preconceived intolerance or hatred of other races.[8,9] Most health care providers would agree that prejudice is incompatible with empathy and objective treatment planning.

OVERVIEW OF CHARACTERISTICS AND HEALTH BELIEFS OF SELECTED MINORITY GROUPS

This overview is not intended to be comprehensive, but should serve as a point of departure for discussion. Remember, there will be many variations within each group described. This is merely an attempt to bring out the salient characteristics and health beliefs of selected minority groups.

Hispanic Americans

The term "Hispanic" was provided by the federal government to identify persons whose ancestry is rooted in Mexico, Puerto Rico, Cuba, Central and South America.[7] Therefore, Hispanics come from many different countries and have a variety of beliefs and values. At the risk of generalizing, Hispanics share some common characteristics as a group. Many Hispanics take pride in their ability to speak and read Spanish. The majority of Hispanics are practicing Roman catholics. Many are in the lower socioeconomic income and live in neighborhoods called barrios.[10] Hispanic Americans have strong family ties and use an extended family system. Godparents (padrinos) often assist with child care or during times of illness. The families are usually patriarchal. The males may subscribe to the macho (machismo) image which implies masculine behavior whereas the female's role is to be the mother of the children, maintain the household, provide understanding and support. In many Hispanic families, the female does not leave home until she gets married. Modesty is another issue that should not be overlooked, especially when interacting with Hispanic women. During physical examinations it is difficult for them to disrobe.[4,11] If the doctor or nurse wishes to talk about family planning or sexual issues, it is best to have the senior male member of the family present.[12] Hispanic Americans also have a strong belief in not revealing personal or family information to strangers. This can be a problem during the initial interview or in treatment planning as many private matters are kept within the family. As a result,

Hispanics are said to be poor candidates for individual psychotherapy but respond better to family therapy. However, in general, Hispanics are reported to have fewer mental health disturbances than the general population.[4] Their physical health status tends to be lower than whites, but is reported to be better than Black Americans.

Hispanics tend to be very emotive people. They are expressive with gestures while involved in group interactions. Females openly express pain, particularly during child birth. Touch is also a strong form of expression among male and female Hispanic Americans. Physical contact such as hugging or holding hands are acceptable behaviors. Lastly, Hispanics are proud of their ethnic music and use food as a form of socialization.[11]

Hispanic Health Beliefs and Practices

Many Hispanic American families use western medicine, but also subscribe to traditional practices such as home remedies (remedios casero) or the use of folk healers (curanderos). Illnesses are often classified according to a system which goes back to ancient times and was used by Hippocrates in his humoral theory of disease. Basically, illnesses are dichotomized into Hot or Cold classifications.[12] According to this theory, the body is regulated by four *humors* (fluids) which are categorized by a combination of hot or cold with wetness or dryness. Most foods, beverages, herbs and medicines are classified as hot or cold (caliente-frio) and are used to restore the body to its natural balance. For example, "hot" conditions are rashes, fever, ulcers, and menstruation. These conditions would be treated with "cold" foods such as fresh vegetables, tropical fruits and milk products. Examples of "cold" conditions are those diseases which bring about an imbalance by stopping the sensory and motor functions of the body. For instance, an earache is due to a cold draft of air entering the ear canal, or rheumatoid arthritis results from external influences of cold. Spicy and acidic foods, herbs or medicines classified as "hot" would be used to treat these ailments.[11]

There are many folk illnesses and disorders recognized by Hispanic Americans that have no counterpart in Western medicine. *Susto* (fright)[11,12,13] is an example of an emotional illness caused by a traumatic experience. It is believed that the soul detaches from the body. The symptoms include withdrawal, listlessness and loss of appetite. This condition would be treated by a curandero (healer) with laying on of hands, prayers, herbs or ritualistic cleansing. *Empacho* is an obstruction of the digestive tract. It is believed to be caused by a ball of undigested food stuff which lodges in the stomach. This usually occurs in children and results in nausea, vomiting, stomachache, fever and perhaps diarrhea. The treatment may include massage of the abdomen and back, herbal teas, prayers and occasional purgatives. *Pasmo*[11,12,13] refers to a tonic spasm of any voluntary muscle resulting from exposure to cold air. Pasmo can also mean stunted growth in children due to parental neglect such as allowing the child to be exposed to extreme temperatures. *Malpuesto*[11,12,13] is the belief that a hex or illness has been put on a person through witchcraft. The "evil put on" may be due to jealousy or envy. Virtually any chronic or unresolved health problem can be attributed to malpuesto. A similar disorder is called *mal de oja*[11,12,13] or "evil eye". This is a magical disorder affecting infants and children. This occurs when a strong person looks at a child but does not touch him. The symptoms include fever, weeping, rashes, vomiting and loss of appetite. The treatment may entail having the person with the strong gaze touch the infant or a ritual of passing an unbroken egg over the body of the infant then placing it under the crib to draw the fever from the child.[13] Another condition affecting infants is *caidade mollera*[12] or fallen fontanel. This is the belief that a sudden removal of the mothers nipple during nursing will cause depression of the soft palate resulting in difficulty in sucking. The symptoms are dehydration, diarrhea, vomiting and restlessness. The treatment includes holding the infant upside down over a pail of hot water or by stimulating the roof of the mouth.

The list of cultural illnesses for Hispanic Americans is very lengthy and goes beyond the scope of this paper.

Indochinese—Southeast Asian Refugees

The Indochinese consist of the South Vietnamese, Laotian, Cambodians and the Hmong. The first large number of Indochinese were admitted to the United States in 1975. These were predominantly professionals, military personnel and government officials who had some close affiliation with the United States. The second wave of refugees arrived in the United States in 1979.[14] These were the less educated and underskilled from more rural areas. It should be remembered that the vast majority of Indochinese in this country are refugees, not immigrants. Many fled their country with little preparation or hopes of returning. The Indochinese speak many different languages and dialects. The extended family is the basic unit of Indochinese culture. The senior male acts as head of the household. Religious beliefs and practices include Buddhism, Confucianism, and Taoist teachings. Many believe that the universal order of the cosmos influences an individual's destiny.[15] The Vietnamese, for example, believe the entire universe is controlled by ever-present deities and spirits. Many worship their ancestors because they believe that the spirits of dead relatives continue to dwell among them and protect their descendants.[16] Indochinese emphasize harmony in social interactions. They have different value orientation to time and many miss appointments or come late. Studies[17,18] have shown that there is a high incidence of psychiatric and psychosomatic problems among the Indochinese refugees. Depression and anxiety are the most common diagnoses for single males between 19 and 35 years of age. Psychosomatic disorders and tension headaches are also common in this population. Indochinese women have been more successful in assimilating to the American culture than the males. This has contributed to material conflict and generational disputes.[1,19]

Health Beliefs and Practices

Indochinese have a variety of beliefs about health and illness. Many of the peasant people believe in natural medicine which is similar to the ancient Greek philosophy of balance (harmony) and the healing power of nature. The hill people (Laotians and Hmong) believe that diseases are caused by the wrath of the gods because of bad conduct by an individual or family member. There is also a Hot-Cold theory relating to the four elements: air, fire, water and earth. Each have an associated characteristic of cold, hot, wet and dry respectively.[19] Balance is restored through the use of herbs, self restraint, meditation and dermabrasive procedures. The dermabrasive procedures are used to alleviate symptoms such as nausea, cough, headache, sore throat, backache and related problems. Rubbing is done with the edge of a coin, piece of bamboo or a spoon. The rubbing abrades the skin leaving minor bruises over the areas of the face, neck, anterior and posterior surfaces of the trunk. In theory, coin rubbing is done to diagnose or to release excessive "air" that is attributed to certain disorders.[19] Other techniques include firmly pinching and pulling on areas of skin and "cupping". Cupping is a method of treatment in which a rounded glass cup from which oxygen has been burnt out, is placed over the primary rami of the spine. As the air in the cup cools, it creates a vacuum and draws the skin upwards. Sometimes the cup is moved up and down leaving a trail of redness on the skin. Indochinese children receiving these treatment may appear to be victims of child abuse.[14]

During pregnancy, Indochinese women take special care to avoid visiting churches and shrines that might be inhabited by evil spirits who could harm them or their unborn children. Many of these women will not leave their houses after dark as the bad spirits are free to roam.[19] It is also believed that if pregnant women look at pictures of healthy children it will in turn cause them to give birth to healthy babies.[19]

Asian Americans

For the purpose of this paper, Asian Americans will include Japanese, Chinese, and Filipino Americans. Each group has its own culture, values, beliefs, attitudes and norms of behavior which have been passed on from generation to generation. Therefore, each group will be discussed individually so some similarities of Asian Americans can be delineated.

Japanese Americans

Approximately 600,000 persons of Japanese ancestry live in the United States with 70% of that population residing in Hawaii and California.[6] The Japanese are a diverse and multi-talented ethnic group who have assimilated well in the United States. They are the healthiest of the ethnic minorities and have achieved a comfortable socioeconomic status.[22] Yip[20] contends that the Japanese were more welcome as immigrants because they were respected for their agricultural skills, frugality and politeness. Kitano[21] has analyzed Japanese Americans according to their generational categories. Each generation is unique and corresponds to significant periods of American history. The first generation to arrive in the U.S. were the *Issei*. They were immigrants who worked diligently on railroads, farms, sawmills and the fishing industry. The second generation, *Nisei* were born before World War II, achieved higher education and a command of the English language. In 1942 the war with Japan intensified hostile feelings towards Japanese Americans and many were evacuated to remote relocation camps until the war ended. *Sansei,* the third generation, continued to increase their education, economic security and to find appropriate employment opportunities. The *Yonsei,* are the fourth and current generation. The third and fourth generations have largely departed from traditional Japanese customs and 50% are married to non-Japanese persons.[21] As a group, half of the Japanese Americans are Christians and one half are Buddhists. They are proud people who do not accept institutional charity.

Japanese Health Beliefs and Practices

In the Japanese communities, mental illness, disfiguring physical disabilities and congenital deformities are viewed as an embarrassment and are met with isolation. The traditional Japanese health belief is rooted in the Shinto religion which holds, by nature, that humans are inherently good. Evil is caused by outside spirits who punish humans who have succumbed to temptation. Health is achieved through balance and harmony. Cleanliness is important due to their belief that disease can be caused by contact with polluting agents. Body odor in Japan, is regarded as a symptom of disease.[22] Japanese health practices are based on the concept of balance, prevention, and cleanliness. Balance is achieved through a diet of fresh sea food, meat and vegetables. Japanese use massage to alleviate tension and sore muscles. Shiatsu is a Japanese style of acupressure which utilizes deep pressure, stretch and equilibrium responses for health maintenence. Martial arts and movement exercises are used to foster physical strength and internal homeostasis.

Chinese Americans

There are approximately 806,027 persons of Chinese ancestry in the United States.[6] The Chinese are stereotyped as being mysterious and quiet with a culture that is exotic.[23] Chinese Americans have migrated from different parts of China and speak many different dialects. Chinese immigration began in 1849 with the California Gold Rush. Many of the immigrants were Cantonese, male, poor and uneducated. Chinese worked long hours for low wages in mining, farming, fishing and railroad construction. Today Chinese

Americans have gained many educational and occupational achievements. However, many Chinese Americans still feel the sting of individual discrimination.[24] Many Chinese inhabit Chinatowns where the job market is limited, living conditions are overcrowded and the chances of upward mobility are reduced.

Chinese Health Beliefs and Practices

Chinese values, behaviors and attitudes are influenced by their philosophical and religious teachings. Many Chinese Americans have internalized the teachings of Taoism, Confucianism and Buddhism which are called the Great Traditions.[25] Given this philosophical base, the Chinese have developed their guiding principles for morality, behavior and science. Some of the values underlying Chinese behavior are benevolence, self respect, social reciprocity, self control, loyalty and righteousness.[24]

Traditional Chinese medicine is based on the theory of Yin and Yang and the Five Elements.[26] Yin (negative, weak, dark, cold, feminine) and Yang (positive, strong, bright, warm, masculine) are diametrically opposed. This dichotomy of Yin/Yang also applies to organs and other functions of the body. The Yin organs are located above the diaphragm, they are solid (Tsang) and include the heart, liver, spleen, lungs, kidney and adrenal glands. The Yang organs are located below the diaphragm, They are hollow (Fu) and include the stomach, gall bladder, urinary bladder and the intestines. Anytime there is an imbalance between Yin and Yang organ functions will be impeded or stimulated causing illness.

The theory of the Five Elements (wu hsing) was derived from empirical observations of nature.[26,27] Chinese scholars codified the relationships among the elements wind, earth, fire, metal and water with nature and various organ systems of the body. Each element has the power to activate or be depressed by the forces of another. It is believed that stimulation to specific sites on the body (acupoints) can activate an innate life energy called Chi (Qi) which moves along pathways called meridians to augment or suppress internal organs. Therefore, acupuncture, acupressure, moxibustion are techniques applied to focal points along meridians to reestablish the balance between Yin and Yang. Traditional Chinese folk medicine also embraces the concept of "wind" and "poison". "Wind" (feng) is a noxious substance that enters the body causing dysfunction. For example exposure to cold is believed to cause arthritis, digestive disorders or cerebrovascular accidents. "Poison" (Tu) describes disease conditions obtained from contaminated foodstuffs or is the result of an endogenous part of the body turning poisonous. Malignant tumors or gangrene are examples of poison (Tu) disorders.[26,27]

Filipino Americans

There are approximately 340,000 Filipino Americans in the United States.[6] The immigration patterns for Filipinos started in 1765 in Louisiana. Since 1965 when the immigration quota system was liberalized, Filipinos have come to the United States in sizable numbers. The Philippines is an archipelago of about 7000 islands. Thus, there are many cultural variations and diversities within the Filipino culture. The regional differences have given rise to numerous Filipino languages.

As a group, Filipinos are very family oriented. Interdependency among family members and respect towards the elderly are highly valued. Many Filipinos are devout catholics and favor the "baha la na" philosophy. This is a fatalistic view of life based on the belief that God's will and supernatural forces control the entire universe. Another trait of Filipino Americans is the emphasis on social acceptance in all human interactions. Filipinos will often avoid direct expressions of conflict. For example, if the therapist imposes an activity that is not appropriate, the Filipino would probably concede gracefully; a concept called pakikisama. At the same time, the Filipino may want to preserve his self-esteem (amor proprio) and would not want to bring shame (hiya) to his family's honor. These values are often misunderstood by health care professionals. The health professional may view the Filipino as indecisive, passive or undependable. Many times, if a Filipino disagrees he may use a "go between" person to iron out the differences.[27]

Filipino Health Beliefs and Practices

Filipino health practices may include concepts of flushing, heating and protection. Flushing is done when it is believed the body contains impurities. A system to stimulate vomiting, perspiration or flatus is used. Heating is done to support the belief that hot and cold qualities must be balanced in the body. Frequent hot baths may be prescribed for an excessive amount of cold. Protection is used to guard against supernatural illnesses. The wearing of ampules, rosaries or religious articles are believed to drive evil forces away.[20,27]

Major Similarities Among Asians

Traditional Asian Americans may subscribe to four major values: (1) Filial Piety, (2) Shame, (3) Self-Control and (4) Social Reciprocity.[15] *Filial piety* basically means the family comes first and the individual comes last. Obedience to parents and preservation of the family's good name is highly regarded. *Shame* may be called Haji (Japanese), face (Chinese) or Hiya (Filipino). This value is derived from the principle of honor, conforming to a code of behavior and fullfillment of obligation. If a Family member does not meet his obligations or exhibits undesirable behavior, he/she will bring shame on the family name. The expression to "save face" describes the behavior of going around situations that may bring conflict. *Self control* or inconspiciousness is also highly valued among Asians. As children, traditional Asians are taught to control their emotions, show patience and perseverance. For example, the Asian patient may not complain when experiencing pain. Because of their quiet behavior, Asians have been called the silent minority.[23]

Social reciprocity is another value honored by Asian Americans. Social reciprocity is expressed in kind words or symbolic gifts as a gesture of wealth or kindness. The Asian patient may wish to reciprocate to the therapist as a gesture of appreciation for services rendered. Rejection of such a gift may offend as it is a token of respect and retribution.[23,26,27]

Black Americans

According to the 1980 census, there are 26,488,218 Blacks in the United States.[6] Black Americans have had a unique experience in that their initial migration to the United States was due to slavery. Much has been written about the social injustices and inadequacies in health care for Black Americans.[28] In short, low income Blacks have found it difficult to avail themselves of costly health care services in the United States.

Black culture is very diverse and an extension of traditions found in the African continent. Cole[29] has outlined four distinctive lifestyles among Black Americans: the street, down-home, militant and upward bound. Each lifestyle has distinct behavioral character-istics and beliefs. Llorens[30] has elaborated on the child rearing practices and health care behavior of Black Americans. According to Llorens, the Black child is born into a society that is culturally alien and rejecting of them. To maintain ingroup solidarity, some Blacks have developed a stylized, rhythmic and spontaneous dialect. Black dialect probably originated during slavery. Slave traders tried to prevent West Africans from communicating with each other by mixing up members of various tribes on ships during their passage to the United States. As a result, the Blacks who spoke two different languages developed a simplified language called Pidgin. This language enabled the Africans to communicate and socialize without the traders understanding their messages. The children of the parents who spoke Pidgin developed a more complete language called Creole.[28]

Black Health Beliefs and Practices

Black American folk medicine believes that illnesses are either "natural" or "unnatural".[31] Natural illnesses are caused by nature's forces such as weather conditions, bad food or water. Unnatural illnesses are brought about by evil forces such as hoodoo, voodoo, witchcraft, rootwork or hexes. Urban Blacks may not subscribe to these beliefs. Baker[32] suggests that stressful socioeconomic circumstances have been attributed as causes of disorders among Blacks in urban areas. For instance, the high prevalence of hypertension among Blacks could be related to stress. Many urban Black Americans place credence in the church as a means of stress reduction and for health maintenance. Saunders reports that church-based hypertension programs have been very successful in urban Black communities.[33]

In Southern geographic regions of the United States, Blacks may believe in a condition called "high blood".[31] High blood does not imply high blood pressure but high blood volume due to over-indulgence of rich food and red meat. Strokes are sometimes attributed to high blood. The folk treatment for this condition is to ingest astringent substances such as vinegar, lemon juice, epsom salts and brine. Jackson[34] has reported a condition called "low blood" which is just the opposite and indicates low blood volume.

To correct this problem, the individual would ingest red meat and rich foods.

Jordan[35] has described three cultural healers in Black American culture. They are described as the "old lady", one who has knowledge of herbs, "the spiritualist", one who has a gift from God for healing; and "the priest", one who has skills in voodoo. When the Black American enters the health care system it is usually a last resort. Thomas[36] states that Blacks exhibit more "paranoid responses" than other patients, resulting in hostility that causes stress for health professionals. The white therapist cannot know how the Black patient feels. The prevalence of racism in America has made some Black Americans deeply suspicious of the white majority. The therapist should be genuine and use a formal approach with the Black American patient.

DEFINING CULTURE AND COMMUNICATION

When two people from different cultures try to transmit information, it is called intercultural communication. Many times, the cultural differences between individuals act as a barrier to communication.

The term "culture" has been defined extensively. Kroeber and Kluckhohn[37] identified 164 definitions of culture. Paul[38] simply defines culture as a "blueprint for social living." This "blueprint" distinguishes one community from another and is passed on from one generation to another.

Culture influences our values, beliefs and perceptions of life. Levine[39] compares culture to a filter which colors the patient's perception along with the degree of involvement in the treatment planning process. The occupational therapist should never assume that his/her own view of life will be similar to those who are from a different cultural background. The success of treatment planning depends on the patient's acceptance and understanding of the goals the therapist wishes to achieve. Therapists are frequently involved in promoting change in patient behavior. The therapist's goals may be culturally rooted in the white middle class value system and not acceptable to the ethnic minority patient. Developing cultural sensitivity requires the willingness to learn about another's culture. The process of learning that takes place between two individuals is contingent upon the communication process. As previously mentioned, intercultural communication occurs when two people from different cultural backgrounds attempt to transmit or receive messages. Intercultural communication requires a sharing of beliefs, attitudes, values, language, touch, use of time, space, forms of expression, religion, myths and social relationships.[40] Much has been written about the components of communication. Porter and Samovar[40] have identified eight components of communication which are (1) source, (2) encoding, (3) message, (4) channel, (5) receiver, (6) decoding, (7) receiver response and (8) feedback. According to Porter and Samovar, these components are only a partial list of factors which transpire during a communication event. Needless to say, communication breakdowns can occur anywhere along the chain of events that make up the communication process.

BASIC TECHNIQUES OF COMMUNICATION

This section will suggest some basic points to consider in the communication process involved in treatment planning.

Interview

In most clinical situations, the first stage of treatment planning is a formal or an informal interview. During the interview, the therapist will try to obtain relevant information about the patient. The interview process also allows the therapist to become more personally acquainted with the individual, to develop a rapport and establish some impression for treatment strategies. Language and nonverbal communication are very important at this phase of treatment planning. If the patient cannot speak or understand English, the therapist should obtain the services of an interpreter. Most health care facilities will have a list of interpreters in the Personnel Office or through the Volunteer Services. The therapist should talk with the interpreter before the interview and clarify the definitions of medical terminology. During the interview, the therapist should use short sentences and concepts that would be understood by the patient if he spoke the same language. The position and distance between the interpreter, therapist and patient is important. The interpreter should be next to the patient, facing the therapist. The therapist should talk to the patient, not the interpreter. Direct eye contact with the patient depends on his cultural background. For example, Mexican Americans will expect eye contact and perhaps some small talk on an informal basis. For many Asian Americans, especially Indochinese, direct eye contact may be considered impolite. In this case, therapists may find it helpful to direct their gaze towards the side of the patient. Black Americans will have different responses to eye contact. Southern Blacks may look down and away from the therapist. Urban blacks perceive wandering eyes as "cut eye" which is felt to be an insult during conversation. The therapist should use a calm and gentle manner to convey the sense of sincerity. Increased voice volume may promote anxiety and disrupt the communication process. The therapist should ask one question at a time and allow the patient and interpreter to formulate a response. Some cultures are indirect in answering a question. Their first responses may only be a vague approximation of their thoughts. Furthermore, in some cultures it is appropriate to think out loud before arriving at an answer. The therapist should look for subtle cues of body language. The Indochinese for instance may say "yes" to most questions. The therapist should phrase questions in such a way that they require some elaboration. Whenever possible, use male interpreters with male patients and female interpreters with female patients. In some Asian cultures, the young female would not normally ask personal questions of an older male. Quesada[41] suggests that differences in social status creates additional communication problems between white middle class health professionals and poor Mexican Americans. According to Quesada, Mexican Americans have a need for paternalistic dependence and develop patron-peon relationships for many activities. For example, the therapist may be regarded as the patron and the Mexican would expect the customary sensitivity to their needs. If the Mexican American feels that he is not getting mutual respect (dignidad) he will usually seek out a curandero (folk healer) for therapy.

Time Factors

The use of time is another element to consider in treatment planning. Hall[42] has observed that cultures use time in two different fashions. There is monochronic time used by industrialized nations where there is reliance upon efficiency, schedules and prompt delivery of services. The second is polychronic time which is observed by so-called third world nations where efficiency is not a factor and customs and human interactions prevail. Therefore, immigrants from underdeveloped nations may abide by polychronic time and not understand why the American therapist is so task oriented. This can put the therapist in an untenable position when trying to schedule treatment sessions. One strategy to deal with patients on polychronic time, is to anticipate that they will be late and schedule the treatment sessions 20 or 30 minutes early. If the patients do arrive near the scheduled time they can be occupied with orientation material or be taken to a section of the clinic where they can begin some self-instructional activities. In any case, it is important for the therapist to set up a free flowing system of scheduling that allows for an informal adherence to time. In addition, many minority patients view the health professional as an authority figure. In their culture, it is more acceptable for them to wait for the person in authority.

Touch

Touch is a transcultural form of communication. Therapists in our society are designated "touchers" by virtue of their profession. Health professionals, hair dressers and tailors are accorded the permission to touch in our culture. During the interview with a non-English speaking patient, selective use of touch by the therapist can be a beneficial way of communicating support and approval. Mason[43] suggests a pat on the shoulder or arm or placing one's hand on the patients hand are acceptable areas to touch. A gentle touch is associated with concern while a firm touch with assurance.

Space

The use of space in intercultural communication will vary from culture to culture. For most Americans, personal distance (life space) is about 18 inches to 4 feet while social distance is about 4 feet to 12 feet.[42] For the therapist it is important to recognize that zones do exist across cultures, and they have definite boundaries and associations within a culture.

During intercultural communication the patient may speak in "broken" English. By virtue of trying to learn English, the patient is attempting to gain assimilation into our culture. It is important to listen to *what* is being said, not *how* it is being said. Patients of Ethnic minorities may speak in dialects, have an accent or speech impediment. It is helpful to concentrate on the message and ask yourself the question: "What is he saying that I need to know?" Therapists should not tune out ideas and health beliefs that do not match their belief systems. An understanding of the patient's culture, health beliefs and practice will augment the treatment planning process.

Most patients of ethnic minority will respond best to a polite and formal approach. It is best to use surnames unless asked to do otherwise. The therapist should refrain from using jargon or colloquialisms as the ethnic minority patient may only understand formal English.

CONCLUSION

The population of the United States is rapidly changing. The influx of ethnic minority patients in the health care delivery system has brought new challenges for occupational therapists. In order to provide quality care that is equal for all, it is important to learn as much as is possible about the culture, health beliefs and practices of the patients we serve. The therapist's knowledge of the patient's belief system impacts upon the treatment planning process. Each ethnic group has its own unique culture but individual variations will occur within each group. The key to better understanding comes from the communication process. The occupational therapist with an understanding of cultural influences on behavior is better prepared to meet the challenge.

REFERENCES

1. Rudov, M, Santangelo, N: *Health Status of Minorities and Low-Income Groups.* U.S. Department of Health, Education and Welfare, Washington, D.C., U.S. Government Printing Office, Pub. No. (HRA) 79-627, 1979

2. Public Health Reports, Supplement to Public Health/Preventing Disease, Sept.-Oct., 3–5, 1983

3. U.S. Department of Commerce, Bureau of the Census: *Current Population Reports:* Population Characteristics, Persons of Spanish Origin in the United States. Series 361:20, 1981

4. Murillo-Rhode, I: Cultural sensitivity in the care of the hispanic patient. *WashStJN—* Special Supplement. 25–32, 1979

5. *Refugee Reports* Office of Refugee Resettlement, U.S. Department of Health and Human Services. Washington, D.C.: 4:16, 1983

6. United States Department of Commerce, *1980 Census of Population,* Subject reports,

Japanese, Chinese and Filipinos in the United States. U.S. Super. of Documents, Washington, D.C.

7. U.S. Department of Commerce, Bureau of Census,: *Age, Sex, Race and Spanish Origin of the Population by Regions, Divisions and States,* Washington, D.C., PC80–51–1, 1980

8. Ruhly, S: *Intercultural Communication.* Chicago, Science Research Associates, Inc., 1982

9. Porter, R.E.: An Overview of Intercultural Communication. In L.A. Sanovar and R.E. Porter (eds.) *Intercultural Communication: A Reader,* Belmont, Ca. Wadsworth Inc. 3–18, 1972

10. McGinnis, M, Green, L: *Strategies for Promoting Health for Specific Populations:* U.S. Department of Health and Human Services, Washington, D.C. U.S. Government Printing Office Pub. 81–50169, 1981

11. Sillen, R: Multi-Cultural Program Manual. Santa Clara Valley Medical Center, San Jose, CA. Multi-Cultural Awareness Training Program 7–15, 1982

12. Currier, R: The hot-cold syndrome and symbolic balance in Mexican and Spanish American folk medicine, In Martinez, R. (ed.) *Hispanic Culture and Health Care: Fact, Fiction, Folklore,* St. Louis: C.V. Mosby, 1978

13. Ahumada-Monrroy, L: Nursing care of roza-latino patients, Orque, M, Block, B, and Ahumada Monrroy, L. (eds.): *In Ethnic Nursing Care: A Multicultural Approach,* St. Louis: C.V. Mosby, 1983

14. Catanzaro, A, Moser, R.J: Health status of refugees from Vietnam, Laos and Cambodia. *JAMA* 247: 1303–1308, 1982

15. Chang, B: *Asian-American Patient Care:* In Transcultural Health Care Menlo Park: Addison Wesley Pub. Co., 1981

16. Schreiber, J, Homiak, J: *Ethnicity and Medical Care,* Cambridge, Massachusetts, Harvard University Press, 1981

17. Smith-Santopietro, M, Lynch, B: What's behind the "inscrutable mask" *RN* 33:55–61, 1981

18. Robinson, C: *Special Report:* Physical and Emotional Health Care Needs of Indochinese Refugees, Indochinese Refugee Action Center, Washington, D.C., 1980

19. Orque, M: Nursing care of South Vietnamese patients In Orque, M, Block, B, Mhumada Monrroy, (eds): *Ethnic Nursing Care,* St. Louis, C.V. Mosby, 1983

20. Yip, B, Lim, H, Fung, V: *Understanding the Pan Asian Client.* San Diego, Ca. Union of Pan Asian Communities, 1978

21. Kitano, H: *Japanese Americans: The Evolution of a Subculture.* 2nd ed. Englewood Cliffs, M.J: Prentice-Hall, Inc., 1976

22. Sato, H, Takano, J: Nursing care of Japanese American patients, In Orque, M, Black, B, Ahumada-Monrroy (eds): *Ethnic Nursing Care,* St. Louis, C.V. Mosby, 1983

23. Maydovich, M: Asian americans-quiet americans? In H.A. Johnson (ed.) *Ethnic American Minorities,* New York, R.R Bowker Co. 71–132, 1976

24. Lee, R: *The Chinese in the United States of America, Hong Kong,* Hong Kong University Press, 1960

25. Beau, G: *Chinese Medicine,* New York, Avon Books, 1972

26. Fung, Y: *A Short History of Chinese Philosophy.* New York, The Free Press, 1961

27. Sue, S, Wagner, N: *Asian Americans Psychological Perspectives.* Palo Alto, Ca. Science and Behavior Books, 1973

28. Blaimer, R: Black culture: Myth or Reality? In P. Rose (ed), *Americans From Africa: Old Memories,* Chicago, Atherton Press, 1970

29. Cole, J: Culture: Negro, Black and Nigger, The Black Scholar, June 1970

30. Llorens, L: Black culture and child development, *Am J. Occup. Ther.* 25, 1971

31. Snow, L: Folk medical beliefs and their implications for care of patients: A review based on studies among black americans, *Ann Int Med* 81:82–96, 1974

32. Baker, A, Cook, G: Stress, adaptation and the Black individual; implications for nursing education. *J Nurs Ed,* 22:237–242, 1983

33. Saunders, E, Dong, W: A role for churches in hypertension management, *Urban Health* 12:49–52, 1983

34. Jackson, J: Urban Black America. In Harwood, A. (ed) *Ethnicity and Medical Care,* Cambridge Mass., Harvard Press 37–129, 1981

35. Jordan, W: Voodoo medicine. In R.A. Williams (ed): *Textbook of Black Related Diseases,* New York, McGraw-Hill Inc. 715–738, 1975

36. Thomas, D: Black American Patient Care. In Henderson, G, Primeaux, M, (eds.): *Transcultural Health Care,* Menlo Park, Ca. Addison-Wesley Pub. Co. 209–223, 1981

37. Kroeber, A, Kluckhohn, C: Culture—*A Critical Review of Concepts and Definitions.* New York. Random House, Vintage Books, 1952

38. Paul, B: The role of beliefs and customs in sanitation programs. *Am J Occ Ther* 48(11):1502–1506, 1958

39. Levine, R: The cultural aspects of home care delivery. *Am J Occ Ther* 38, 728–737, 1984

40. Samovar, L, Portes, R: *Intercultural Communication: A reader,* Belmont Ca., Wadsworth Pub. Co., 1985

41. Quesada, F: Language and communication barriers for health delivery to a minority group. *Social Science and Medicine.* 10:323–327, 1976

42. Hall, E: *Beyond Culture.* Garden City, N.Y., Anchor Books, 1976

43. Mason, A, Pratt, J: Touch. *Nursing Times.* June, 999–1001, 1980

Ethnic/Racial Considerations
in Occupational Therapy:
A Survey of Attitudes

Kathryn A. Skawski

ABSTRACT. Examination of the occupational therapy literature related to cultural factors in treatment inspired investigation into the levels of cultural awareness of currently practicing therapists. White, black, Asian-American, Puerto Rican and Mexican-American therapists were selected to receive a questionnaire involving factors that encourage or discourage cultural sensitivity in the clinical setting. Some of the results of the study will be reported and discussed.

Few American occupational therapists would assert that today's society consists of a homogenous population. Yet the popular conception of a ''melting-pot'' perpetuates the myth that all ethnic and racial minorities have been steadily assimilating into the dominant middle-class American culture. This notion bears scant resemblance to the reality of the myriad of different subcultures currently existing in the United States.

The sheer variety of subcultures found in this country raises the possibility of problematic interaction between individuals of dissimilar cultural backgrounds. Successful intercultural communication is dependent upon an awareness of and respect for differences in values, customs and language patterns.[1] As a service dependent upon successful communication for efficacy, health care is particularly liable to failure in this area.[2-5] Often, the delivery of medical and therapeutic services follows a predetermined format that fails to address the value orientation and social framework of a particular client.

Kathryn A. Skawski is an occupational therapy graduate student at the University of Puget Sound currently completing fieldwork assignments.

This paper appears jointly in *Sociocultural Implications in Treatment Planning in Occupational Therapy* (The Haworth Press, Inc., 1987) and in *Occupational Therapy in Health Care*, Volume 4, Number 1 (Spring 1987).

37

In response to the growing demands of a multicultural population, various branches of the health professions have begun reassessing the needs of culturally-distinct clients. Physicians, nurses, counselors and occupational therapists have contributed to a greater understanding of the impact of cultural background upon the provision of health care.[2-7,9-25] In the past two decades, coursework in the cultural aspect of illness and disability has been added to curricula of health professions.[6,7]

The question of the relevance of culture to health care will continue as an important concern to all health service providers. The affirmation of ethnic and racial pride that had its roots in the Civil Rights Movement has been firmly established. Also, the continued influx of large numbers of immigrants from disparate cultures shows no signs of abating, immigration quotas notwithstanding. In 1982 alone, 626,000 Indochinese refugees and 125,000 Cubans entered the United States.[8]

Given that cultural sensitivity is an issue in health care—what implications does this fact have for the field of occupational therapy? Most experienced therapists agree that the value orientations related to productivity, self-maintenance and leisure are culturally specific to some degree. However, the relationship of cultural background to treatment planning is not well articulated in the occupational therapy literature. Evaluation and assessment of functioning are largely based on the sociocultural norms of a white middle-class population.

At the present time, it is the therapist's task to respond and adapt to the diverse population presented in everyday practice. It is likely that most practicing therapists will encounter clients from cultures with value orientations that reject the type of therapy routinely offered. Awareness of and respect for varying cultural norms—the therapist's as well as the client's—will facilitate the therapeutic process and meet occupational therapy's goal of holistic treatment.

REVIEW OF THE LITERATURE

The development of a cultural consciousness in the field of health care is inseparable from the social history of the United States. Dodd[4, p. 1] suggested that "The period of the 1960's in the United States also marked a kind of cultural awakening." In support of this contention is the fact that in 1964, Sanchez was among the first in the literature to call attention to the white middle-class bias of the "helping professions." He proposed that occupational therapy should incorporate the patient's cultural background into treatment in order for therapy to be effective.

During the volatile era of the Civil Rights Movement, however, the issue of culture in health care appears to have taken a back seat to the more pressing concerns of discrimination in education, employment and economic opportunity. Only after some discernible gains were consolidated in these areas did attention return to the persistent problem of the inability of many health care professionals to respond effectively to the needs of minority clients. This trend is reflected in the literature in general as well as specifically in the occupational therapy literature. After Sanchez' article in 1964, no other discussion of this issue appeared in the occupational therapy literature until 1971.

As the most visible and vocal subculture, black Americans became the primary focus of literature related to cultural differences. Llorens[10] described the types of lifestyles found in the black community and their impact upon child development. An increasing awareness of cultural diversity and divergent values seems to be reflected in subsequent research.

In 1972 Klavins[11, p. 177] posed the still unanswered question: "As a profession (OT) which deals with the work and play behaviors of a great variety of people, how much do we know of the cultural influences they experience?" The acknowledgement of a weakness in cultural awareness led to examination of the relationship of racial similarity of client and therapist to therapeutic success. Banks[12] and Gardner[13] found that black counselors were more effective with black clients than were white counselors. According to Allen[14, p. 58] "black clients often doubt white therapists' capacity to understand them." Danek and Lawrence,[15] however, reported that black and white counselors were equally successful with black rehabilitation clients.

Failure to establish therapeutic rapport has also been reported with Asian-American clients and white therapists. Tsui and Schultz[16] described adaptations in clinical style that can be made by non-Asian therapists in order to establish a successful therapeutic relationship with Asian-American clients such as appropriate self-disclosure and slower pace of treatment. Sue[17] and Yamamoto[18] have also contributed to research on the dynamics of counseling Asian clients.

Kleinman, et al.[119, p. 251] proposed the concept of a "clinical social science capable of translating concepts from cultural anthropology into clinical language for practical application.'' Parry[20] discussed anthropological terminology in terms of differing views of diagnosis and treatment in physical therapy. The specialty of medical anthropology represents a mainstream acceptance of the importance of cultural considerations in the treatment of illness.

The current literature discussing cultural sensitivity in health care reflects the transformed attitude of the past few decades. Acceptance of the importance of this issue is assumed and the trend is toward providing specific information that will aid the clinician in providing treatment to all types of clients. It is vital to note that the purpose is not to replace old stereotypes with new ones, but rather, to provide information regarding possible cultural traits that may aid the clinician in providing treatment to clients of dissimilar cultures. The degree to which the individual may be acculturated to white middle-class values must always be taken into consideration.

The rapidly expanding Hispanic population in the United States provides a good example of a diverse ethnic group reflecting large disparities in acculturation. Length of residence in the United States, fluency in English and physical proximity to the country of origin all affect the rate and degree of assimilation and consequently which traditional cultural values may or may not be retained.

Murillo-Rohde[21] has shown how folk medicine plays an important role in the Hispanic view of illness and that the hot-cold theory often has a significant impact upon treatment. Gibson[22] reported on Hispanic cultural values such as the significance of the family and the phenomenon of biculturalism.

Another visible subculture is the large number of Southeast Asian refugees who have arrived in the United States within the past ten years. Although many have assimilated rapidly into American culture, traditional beliefs and practices still exist among many of these immigrants. Nguyen[3] described a disturbing incident of a misinterpretation of a Vietnamese folk remedy that resulted in a mistaken charge of child abuse. The Vietnamese parent was jailed and subsequently committed suicide as a result of the shame connected with the incident.

Dixon, et al.[23] described a movement in Alaska to provide ''culturally-appropriate'' health care to Alaskan natives. Levine[24] used a case study of an Italian-American client to demonstrate the effect of cultural factors upon occupational therapy services in a home setting.

Despite the acknowledged development of a cultural consciousness in health care, however, many would assert that there are health professionals who have not progressed in their ability to incorporate cultural awareness into treatment. Jenkins and Ames[23, p. 59] reported that less than half of black disabled students surveyed "felt that service providers helped them reach their potential or saw them as worthy people."

PURPOSE OF THE STUDY

The purpose of this study was to explore the levels of cultural awareness and sensitivity among currently practicing occupational therapists. The holistic nature of occupational therapy encourages practicing therapists to respond to all the needs of a client— including sociocultural traits that may affect treatment.

It was anticipated that varying levels of social experience and occupational therapy curriculum content would contribute to the development of an awareness of the importance of cultural considerations in the treatment process. It was also anticipated that experience with diverse patient populations would increase the cultural awareness of the clinician.

METHODOLOGY

The subjects selected for this study included white, black, Asian-American, Puerto Rican and Mexican-American occupational therapists registered with AOTA in New York and California. All black, Puerto Rican, Mexican-American and Asian-American therapists (from New York only) were selected due to the relatively small numbers in these groups. Twelve percent of the white occupational therapists were randomly selected from each state. Forty percent of the Asian-American therapists in California were also randomly selected. This relatively large proportion was selected in order to account for the diversity of the Asian-American population in California.

The measuring instrument used was a questionnaire containing structured and open-ended items. All therapists received the same questionnaire with a copy of the cover letter.

Content validity of the questionnaire was established by consultation with a medical anthropologist and a sociologist experienced in race relations. Then a pilot study was conducted using fifteen subjects to assess clarity of the questionnaire. Responses received indicated no problems with clarity.

RESULTS AND DISCUSSION

Of the 830 mailed questionnaires, 144 useable responses were received—indicating a response rate of 17%. Because AOTA does not release mailing labels based on ethnic and racial origin, a blind mailing was done through AOTA and a second mailing was not feasible.

Responses received from Puerto Rican and Mexican-American therapists were not included in analysis due to the small number of responses received from these two groups. Analysis was based on responses from white, black and Asian-American therapists.

The low response rate of this study limits generalization, but the geographical and ethnic/racial diversity of the subjects provides valuable information regarding the levels of cultural awareness for the therapists surveyed. Comments given by the therapists of varying ethnic and racial backgrounds illustrate attitudes regarding the role culture plays in occupational therapy delivery. Twenty-five percent of respondents indicate that they felt unprepared for the client populations encountered after graduation.

Significantly more black therapists perceived themselves as prepared to deal with the ethnic/racial characteristics of the client population that they encountered after graduation than did Asian-American therapists ($x^2 = 7.51$ p = .01). No significant differences for this variable were found between white and black therapists or between white and Asian-American therapists, as illustrated in Table 1.

Another measure of culture awareness is the extent to which an individual identifies with his or her own cultural background. A significantly greater number of black therapists indicated strongly embracing their own culture than did white therapists ($x^2 = 17.69$ p < .001) as seen in Table 2. A significant difference was also found to exist for this variable with black therapists reporting more interest in their backgrounds than did Asian-American therapists ($x^2 = 7.86$ p = .005). White therapists were the only group in which 10% of

Table 1

Therapist origin and perception of preparation

	n	Prepared	Not Prepared	No Response
Black	(19)	89.5%*	5.3%	5.2%
White	(86)	66.3%	30.3%	3.4%
Asian	(21)	56.5%*	34.8%	8.7%

$x^2 = 7.51$ $p = .01$

Table 2

Therapist origin and interest in culture

	n	Strongly Embrace	Enjoy Some Parts	Not Interested
Black	(19)	68.4%**	31.6%	0%
Asian	(23)	39.1%*	60.9%	0%
White	(88)	27.0%*	61.8%	10%

*$x^2 = 17.69$ $p < .001$
**$x^2 = 7.68$ $p = .005$

the respondents indicated no interest at all in their ethnic or cultural background.

An additional method of measuring cultural awareness and sensitivity is to examine perceptions of the therapist's and the client's background and how these factors affect the treatment process. The respondents were presented with two open-ended questions.

a. How can the cultural background of the *client* enhance or interfere with the treatment process?

b. How can the cultural background of the *therapist* enhance or interfere with the treatment process?

For analysis responses were coded as: (1) Enhance only, (2) Interfere only, (3) Both enhance and interfere, (4) Neither. The first two categories were selected for analysis as they represent opposing attitudes. Analysis of responses to these two questions was done in relation to the therapist's identification of the ethnic/racial characteristics of his or her current client population. There were no differences in composition of client populations. Therefore, the differences found in the responses of white, black and Asian-American therapists to the question of the therapist's versus the client's background cannot be attributed to different ethnic/racial characteristics of client populations.

Black therapists were more likely to describe the therapist's background as enhancing and the client's background as interfering with the treatment process ($x^2 = 6.85$ p $= .01$) as illustrated in Table 3. Asian-American therapists reported that both the therapist's and the client's background were more likely to interfere with treatment than enhance it ($x^2 = 6.56$ p $= .01$). White therapists also indicated interference as more likely for both the client's and the therapist's background.

As indicated above, most therapists responding to the survey indicated that the client's background was more likely to interfere with the treatment process than enhance it. An Asian-American therapist said: "It has, on some occasions, led to a longer time for clients to trust me, because I look so different and some have even

Table 3

Therapist origin, therapist's background/client's background, and treatment (enhance/interfere)

		Enhance treatment		Interfere		
White	Therapist	22.5%	n=20	28.1%	n=25	
	Client	12.4%	n=11	31.5%	n=28	No sig
Black	Therapist	26.3%	n=5	15.8%	n=3	x^2=6.85
	Client	10.5%	n=2	21.1%	n=4	p=.01
Asian	Therapist	13.0%	n=3	30.4%	n=7	x^2=6.56
	Client	0%		17.4%	n=4	p=.01

verbalized concern over my educational background and capability." Several Asian-American therapists raised the issue of difficulty in dealing with veterans of WWII and the Korean War due to hostility on the client's part. A black therapist stated "Some whites that I have encountered are not prepared to receive instruction from a black."

White therapists also made strong statements regarding their perception of clients' cultural backgrounds interfering with the treatment process. "Desire to improve and follow through on therapy programs is better with most white clients." Another therapist remarked "Japanese wives seem very demeaning of their husbands with strokes saying their spouse was now 'just like baby'. Hispanic women with strokes felt they now deserved to be taken care of and often weren't real motivated."

Other white therapists who responded that the client's cultural background may interfere with therapy took responsibility for this interference in identifying how their expectations conflicted with those of their clients. One therapist stated "It does affect the treatment process. They have a different view of ADL, whereas the treatment program is offered from a white middle-class background." Another therapist remarked "WASP's (White Anglo-Saxon Protestant) are geared to be independent, with a strong work ethic—expecting (the same from) other cultures or personalities may interfere with the effectiveness of treatment and its ultimate outcome." One therapist concluded "I think WASP therapists may tend to have a more limited perspective overall."

Another factor which measures levels of cultural awareness is the percentage of therapists who indicated that they felt prepared even though there had been no information regarding culture in their occupational therapy curricula. Analysis revealed a significant difference between prepared therapists who indicated that their occupational therapy curriculum contained this information and those who indicated that it had not ($x^2 = 13.22$ p $<$ .001) as seen in Table 4. The large proportion of therapists who felt prepared even though this issue had not been included in their curricula supports the contention that therapists with a high degree of cultural awareness have obtained this information through social experience related to their own ethnic or racial background.

This conclusion is also supported by the fact that significantly more black therapists felt prepared for cultural diversity. Black therapists indicated a stronger interest in their own culture and they were

Table 4

Perception of preparation and cultural content in curriculum

	n	Prepared	Not Prepared
Cultural content	(36)	31.3%*	13.5%
No cultural content	(97)	67.7%*	81.1%

$x^2 = 13.22$ $p < .001$

more likely to see their own cultural backgrounds as enhancing the treatment process. A black therapist discussing the way in which the therapist's background can enhance the treatment process stated "I believe that the therapist of minority background has a far easier task understanding the cultural background of others, since, by necessity, our sensitivities have been increased. I believe that this may be a much more difficult task for therapists from the majority culture."

Ethnocentrism is a luxury that black therapists cannot afford if they are to survive the socialization process of becoming an occupational therapist. White therapists, however, are not challenged to examine their own attitudes regarding cultural factors because there is an inherent assumption that "everybody does things that way." As one white therapist stated "Foreign therapists are sometimes slow in doing self-care and ADL's as we do it in the U.S.A." Another therapist remarked "I have caught myself saying that patients have sequencing problems if they brush their teeth differently than I do."

CONCLUSION

The results of this study indicate that the relevance of sociocultural factors to treatment has not been adequately stressed in occupational therapy education. The amount of time devoted to this issue in a curriculum indicates to the students its relative importance. Lip service in the classroom can translate to lip service in the clinical setting. The amount of time spent learning treatment theories, however, is worthless, if the therapist is unable to establish a therapeutic relationship in which this information can be utilized.

Occupational therapy's goal of providing holistic treatment implies consideration of sociocultural factors in the treatment process. Therapists of different ethnic and racial backgrounds display varying levels of the cultural awareness and sensitivity necessary for meeting the needs of clients. Most occupational therapists currently practicing in the United States are part of an unquestioning majority. This can negatively affect the provision of health care services to culturally-distinct clients if occupational therapists are not aware of their own values and those of their clients.

Time constraints and language difficulties are just a few of the factors that may discourage cultural sensitivity in the clinical setting. However, attitudes and preconceived perceptions of behavior, impact the provision of therapy. As one respondent stated, "The therapist must be open, non-critical and accepting of everyone he or she treats or he or she has no right to treat that patient."

REFERENCES

1. Dodd CH: *Dynamics of Intercultural Communication*. Dubuque: William C. Brown, 1982

2. Hartog J, Hartog EA: Cultural aspects of health and illness behavior in hospitals. *West J Med* 139:910–916, 1983

3. Nguyen D: Culture shock—A review of Vietnamese culture and its concepts of health and disease. *West J Med* 142:409–412, 1985

4. Clark M: Cultural context of medical practice. *West J Med* 139:806–810, 1983

5. Kim SS: Ethnic elders and American health care—A physician's perspective. *West J Med* 139:885–891, 1983

6. Brodsky CM: Culture and disability behavior. *West J Med* 139:892–897, 1983

7. Stein HF: The culture of the patient as a red herring in clinical decision making: A case study. *Med Anthropol*, 1985

8. U.S. Bureau of the Census, *Statistical Abstracts of the United States*. Washington, D.C., 1984

9. Sanchez V: Relevance of cultural values. *Am J Occup Ther* 17:1–5, 1964

10. Llorens LA: Black culture and child development. *Am J Occup Ther* 25:144–148, 1971

11. Klavins R: Work-play behavior: Cultural influences. *Am J Occup Ther* 26:176–179, 1972

12. Banks WM: The differential effects of race and social class in helping. *J Clin Psych* 28:90–92, 1972

13. Gardner WE: The differential effects of race, education and experience in helping. *J Clin Psych* 28:87–89, 1972

14. Allen IM: Posttraumatic stress disorder among black Vietnam veterans. *Hosp & Comm Psych* 37:55–61, 1986

15. Danek MM, Lawrence RE: Client-counselor racial similarity and rehabilitation outcome. *J Rehab* 48:54–58, 1982

16. Tsui P, Schultz G: Failure of rapport: Why psychotherapeutic engagement fails in the treatment of Asian clients. *Am J Orthopsychiat* 55:561–569, 1985

17. Sue, DW: Eliminating Cultural Oppression in Counseling. In *Human Services for Cultural Minorities*. RH Dana, Editor. Baltimore: University Park Press, 1981

18. Yamamoto J: Therapy for Asian Americans. In *Human Services for Cultural Minorities*. RH Dana, Editor. Baltimore: University Park Press, 1981

19. Kleinman A, Eisenberg L, Good B: Culture, illness and care. *Ann Int Med* 88:251–258, 1978

20. Parry KK: Concepts for medical anthropology for clinicians. *Phys Ther* 64:929–933, 1984

21. Murillo-Rohde I: Cultural sensitivity in the care of the Hispanic patient. *Wa St J Nurs*, 1979

22. Gibson G: Hispanic women: Stress and mental health issues. In *Women Changing Therapy*. JH Robbins, RJ Sugel, Editors. New York: Haworth Press, 1983

23. Dixon M, Myers W, Book P, Nice P: The changing Alaskan experience. *West J Med* 139:917–922, 1983

24. Levine RE: The cultural aspects of home care delivery. *Am J Occup Ther* 38:734–738, 1984

25. Jenkins AE, Ames OC: Being black and disabled: A pilot study. *J Rehab* 49:54–60, 1983

A New Social Perspective on Disability and Its Implications for Rehabilitation

Carol J. Gill, PhD

ABSTRACT. As disabled people become more active and vocal in asserting their rights, they are sharing important information about the experience of disability in our society. In fact, they are challenging the definitions and models of disability traditionally utilized in rehabilitation practice. This paper contrasts the traditional medical model of disability with a new interactional or sociopolitical model. The experience of disability is examined in the context of disabled people's minority group status. Also discussed are the efforts of disabled persons to fashion a positive identity and sense of cultural pride. Arguments are presented for addressing the social aspects of disability in rehabilitation.

It is often said that if you want the most accurate information about something, you should "ask the man who owns one." In the study of physical disability, however, the person who "owns one" is no longer waiting to be asked. People with disabilities are eagerly taking the initiative these days and sharing crucial information which, all too often, professionals have neglected to elicit.

The disability civil rights and consumer self-advocacy movements have gained significant momentum in the past decade. Accordingly, as disabled people achieve success in publicly voicing their needs, they offer eloquent reports of the experience of disability in their lives.[1,2,3,4] They talk about feelings, goals, and concepts. In addition, they are framing new questions and suggest-

Carol J. Gill earned her doctorate in psychology from the University of Illinois, Chicago. She is a practicing clinical psychologist in Los Angeles and is the Acting Director of the Program in Disability and Society at the University of Southern California. She was formerly the Director of Rehabilitation Psychology at Glendale Adventist Medical Center, Glendale, California. Address correspondence to: 4419 Van Nuys Boulevard, Suite 401, Sherman Oaks, CA 91403.

This article appears jointly in *Sociocultural Implications in Treatment Planning in Occupational Therapy* (The Haworth Press, Inc., 1987) and in *Occupational Therapy in Health Care*, Volume 7, Number 1 (Spring 1987).

49

ing innovative ways of looking at disability to guide scientific inquiry and professional practice.

A particularly important recent development is that disabled people have begun to challenge standard definitions and models of disability. Traditionally, disability has been conceptually tied to the medical model. From this perspective, a disability is a structural or functional impairment—a negative deviation from "normal." Disability is located within the individual. The individual, then, is the focus of all corrective or assistive intervention, and the agent of intervention is the health care professional.

A conceptualization of disability which differs significantly from the medical model and which is rapidly gaining adherents among disability experts, is the interactional or socio-political model.[5,6] From this perspective, disability is defined not only by the physical qualities of an individual but also by the corresponding response of the social environment. Disability, in this view, does not reside solely in the individual; rather it derives from the interaction between the individual and society. Furthermore, the correction of disability-related problems is no longer solely the province of health professionals but may also be effected by peer support, political activism, and self-help.

An example may serve to clarify the contrasting emphases of the two models. Suppose a man who uses a wheelchair discovers he is unable to enter a restaurant which has a flight of stairs at the entrance. Applying the medical model, we would attribute his dilemma to the paralysis in his legs. A possible solution would be to secure the help of rehabilitation therapists to teach the man to ascend stairs with crutches. Applying the socio-political model, on the other hand, we might attribute his difficulty to the ill-informed architect who design the building or to society's failure to provide equal access to all citizens. A possible solution would be to consult an advocacy group for guidance in filing a law suit against the restaurant. In one case, a physical intervention is performed on the individual. In the other case, an intervention is chosen to modify society's interaction with the individual.

An advantage of the socio-political model, in contrast to the medical model, is its ability to address the cultural relativity of constructs such as "disability" and "normality." Beatrice Wright[7] illustrates the relativity issue using the example of foot-binding in ancient China. This practice produced structural deviations in women's feet which rendered some unable to walk. To move from place to place, they were carried. We in modern Western society would consider this a disability, not to mention a burden of dependency on others. Yet people of that culture viewed such women as normal, even beautiful.

Another important advantage of the socio-political model is that it reflects most accurately the comprehensive experience of disabled individuals as reported in their own accounts. Increasingly, people with disabilities are identifying themselves as members of a large and largely overlooked minority group. Recent surveys indicate that more than 30 million Americans have some type of disability.[8] The majority live at or below the poverty level. A substantial proportion are unemployed due to job discrimination and many still encounter unequal access to education and community resources. Isolation and interpersonal rejection plague disabled people due to pervasive prejudice regarding disability in our culture. It is not surprising that in interviews and written accounts, disabled individuals repeatedly observe that most of the frustration in their lives derives not from their disabilities but from the handicapping barriers constructed by society.

The notion that people with a wide range of disabilities all belong to a common social group—a minority group—is an innovative concept. Whereas the medical model focuses on discrete diagnostic categories to describe correlates of disability, the new socio-political perspective acknowledges the commonality of disability experiences across diagnostic groups. Disabled people, regardless of medical diagnosis, have begun to acknowledge their common treatment by a society which generally devalues and fears disability. This devaluation and consequent social oppression, they say, results in a shared feeling of what it means to be a disabled person in our culture.

As disabled people recognize and appreciate their shared social experience, this growing group identity forms the foundation of a counter-cultural disability pride movement, analogous historically to the cultural efforts of other minority groups in their search for unity and positive identity.[9] For example, just as other minority groups adopted formerly pejorative terms to infuse them with positive meaning (e.g., "black"), disability-rights groups insist on maintaining control of their own terminology and declare as positive such terms as "disabled." Moreover, many individuals object to any view of disability as inherently negative. They emphasize the rarely acknowledged salutary contributions of disability in their lives: enhanced creativity, sensitivity, inner strength, and the deepening and clarification of values. They criticize what they regard as the rigidity and superficiality of majority cultural values, such as physical perfection, youthfulness, material achievement, and extreme independence.

Increasingly, people with disabilities express pride in the perspective and skills they have developed in living with the dual challenge of disability limitations and social stigma. Some use the term, "disability consciousness," to denote a person's level of awareness of all the factors composing the disability experience, particularly social and political components. A national publication, *Disability Rag*[10] has popularized the phrase "disability cool" to describe the poise and self-possession exhibited by many disabled individuals, not *in spite* of disability but *because* of it.

A growing number of disabled people reject suggestions that they can be perceived more positively when viewed apart from their disabilities. They take issue with societal encouragement to "overcome" their physical differentness. They resent applause for accomplishing goals "despite" disability or hearing they are attractive or likeable "even though" they are disabled. Their argument is that disability has become an integral part of who they are. To reject the disability is to deny an essential building block of identity.

Disability activists are also speaking out against the paternalism and sense of charity society evidences in addressing many disability-rights issues. Some refuse to express gratitude. They assert their full and equal citizenship and point out that equal access would be a current reality if society had not chosen to construct the environment in ways which exclude disabled inhabitants unnecessarily. A university student with a spinal cord injury recently reflected this position, saying she was learning to expect her equal rights without "apologizing for being disabled." Or, as a tee-shirt on sale at a recent disability products show unabashedly proclaimed, "I WANT IT ALL!"

Although not yet universally adopted throughout the disability community, this untraditional perspective is catching fire. Like the trend toward general consumerism, it promises to remain a potent force in the future. If so, it will be impossible to ignore its more serious challenges to the theory and practice of physical rehabilitation.

While there has been a trend toward de-centralizing authority in rehabilitation through treatment team approaches and greater patient/

family involvement in goal-setting, the power of medical "experts" in determining the course of rehabilitation is undeniable. Yet any rehabilitation program which does not also give considerable weight to the social aspects of disability—including the minority status of all disabled individuals—may be failing to fulfill its primary goal: restoring patients to a functional life.

Disability activists charge that the medicalization of rehabilitation harms disabled individuals in several ways. First, viewing disability as a medical problem reinforces society's avoidance of responsibility for accommodating disabled citizens. The man, mentioned previously, who expends all his energy arduously learning to ascend stairs with crutches may never take action to insure that his community becomes more accessible to all persons with disabilities.

Second, when disability is perceived solely as a problem within the individual, negative feelings provoked by the frustrations of daily living can flow in only one direction, inward. The patient's anger and despair are expressed against the self, e.g., "I hate my legs; I hate my body; I'm angry with myself." However, when the social component of disability is acknowledged, a patient can identify justified anger and appropriately turn it outward on handicapping public policies, e.g., "My legs may be paralyzed but I still deserve access to my community."

Third, when rehabilitation services center almost exclusively on goals of physical functioning and normalization, professionals may lose sight of the fact that their patients are complete and complex human beings with goals and interests of their own. To reinforce a patient's natural coping ability, the professional must attend to fundamental human needs, e.g., relationships, sexuality, artistic expression, and recreation.

Rehabilitation staff members are also members of society. They too must ward off the stereotyped thinking about disability which dominates our culture and which characterizes disabled people as weak, child-like, lacking in judgment, and incapable of enjoying life in all the ways that nondisabled people do. Viewing patients in this light violates their sense of self-esteem. It undermines their drive for self-determination and their ultimate potential for functional living.

For rehabilitation to be helpful, it must address the reality of what life is like for disabled persons. If rehabilitation professionals fail to fit their services to the patient's needs, values, and interests, they fail both the patient and their own professional aspirations. Frequently, the first symptom of this is patient non-compliance or poor motivation. However, too few rehabilitation professionals actually possess the requisite knowledge. They study technique and theory. In their work, they meet hundreds of disabled individuals who are ill, or ill-informed. However, they receive all too few glimpses of the quality of life actually existing in the highly functioning disability community. They learn little about the struggles of disabled people to fashion a positive adjustment through confronting society's reluctance to welcome them and recognize them as its own citizens.

Although professionals with a strong investment in the medical model might disagree, rehabilitation is precisely the place where patients need to learn about society's response to disability. Patients rely on rehabilitation to help them understand disability and to prepare them for returning to life in the community. Without a proper balance of physical treatment and realistic social information, rehabilitation professionals cannot enable patients. What good are significant gains in physical functioning without skills to evaluate and address society's treatment of disabled people? What good are increased range of motion and finger dexterity when a patient's morale can be crushed by job discrimination or social rejection?

Rehabilitation is also the place where patients can begin to sift through relevant cultural values in defining their identities as disabled people. They must determine which values are still appropriate and which need critical reassessment. Sometimes at its worst, rehabilitation endorses the very elements of our cultural ethic that reject physical differences among people. Professionals must guard against narrowly and inflexibly defining such goals as physical independence. Disabled people have creatively demonstrated the variety of ways one can be independent, including ways that incorporate elective assistance. Misguided beliefs about what is "best" for patients must not supercede patients' own choices of equally beneficial alternatives.

Living well with a disability is as much art as science. Those individuals who, through practice and creative drive, become accomplished in this art can be duly proud, for it takes considerable strength to cope successfully with both the physical and social realities of any disability. For too long the social or cultural side of the equation had escaped notice. Fortunately, disabled people in characteristic style pioneered the discovery of the complex nature of disability in our society.

It is accurate to say that in finding the missing social components of the disability formula, disabled people found themselves. The socio-political model finally made sense of their experience and facilitated genuine self-acceptance. It remains to be seen whether professionals in the field of rehabilitation will support and embrace these efforts or not. There can be no better ''medicine,'' after all, for the difficulties of disability than self-acceptance. How good it would be if the spark of cultural pride already ignited in the disability community could be nourished, not neglected, in rehabilitation.

REFERENCES

1. Bullard, DG and Knight, SE (eds): *Sexuality and Physical Disability: Personal Perspectives*. St. Louis: CV Mosby Company, 1981

2. Duffy, Y: *All Things Are Possible*. Ann Arbor, MI: AJ Garvin and Associates, 1981

3. Matthews, GF: *Voices From the Shadows*. Toronto: Women's Education Press, 1983

4. Zola, IK: Missing Pieces: *A Chronicle of Living With a Disability*. Philadelphia: Temple University Press, 1982

5. DeJong, G: Defining and implementing the independent living concept, in Crewe, NM and Zola, IK: *Independent Living for Physically Disabled People*. San Francisco: Jossey-Bass, 1983

6. Hahn, H: Disability policy and the problem of discrimination. *Am Beh Sci* 1985:28 (Jan/Feb):293–318

7. Wright, B: *Physical Disability—A Psychosocial Approach*. ed 2. New York: Harper and Row, 1983

8. Bowe, F: *Handicapping America: Barriers to Disabled People*. New York: Harper and Row, 1978

9. Longmore, PK: A note on language and the social identity of disabled people. *Am Beh Sci* 1985:28(Jan/Feb): 419–423

10. *Disability Rag*. Louisville, KY: Advocado Press

Appalachian Values:
Implications
for Occupational Therapists

Anne B. Blakeney, MSOT, OTR

ABSTRACT. Appalachia is a distinct geographic region within the United States and natives of this region live within a separate subculture. Initially, inhabitants of this region shared the values of many other early American settlers. However, in time the relative isolation of this region produced a dichotomy between the way of life in an increasingly technological American society and that found within the slower changing region of Appalachia. Thus, the values of Appalachian people today reflect these continued differences.

Occupational therapists treating patients from Appalachia need to understand the values of this subculture in order to assess their patients accurately and to provide culturally appropriate treatment. This paper presents an overview of Appalachian values, with implications for occupational therapy.

Southern Appalachia, sometimes referred to as the Southern Highlands, extends geographically from the Mason-Dixon line on the north, in a southwesterly direction into northern Georgia and Alabama. It encompasses the mountain regions in the states of Maryland, Virginia, Kentucky, Tennessee, North and South Carolina, Georgia, Alabama, and all of West Virginia. It makes up about one-third of the total area of these states and includes approximately one-third of their total population.[1]

Historically, this region has been continually involved in controversy. As Kentucky writer Harry Caudill has noted, "it has been discovered and rediscovered many times, and what is needed today

Anne B. Blakeney is Assistant Professor, Department of Occupational Therapy, Eastern Kentucky University, Richmond, KY.

This article appears jointly in *Sociocultural Implications in Treatment Planning in Occupational Therapy* (The Haworth Press, Inc., 1987) and in *Occupational Therapy in Health Care*, Volume 4, Number 1 (Spring 1987).

57

are not additional discoveries and revelations but appreciation of what has already been found and written about."[2, p. xiii]

In the 1960's, President Johnson launched his "War on Poverty" and the nation's attention was turned toward areas such as Appalachia. Investigators poured into this region to study, observe, expose, or write about those they came to "uplift." The majority of these individuals usually found whatever they were conditioned to find. "Beauty or ugliness, promise or failure are to an extent in the eyes of the beholders . . . most who came saw primarily the poverty, the ugliness, and the hopelessness. None would deny that these are there, even though some observers found also beauty and integrity and joy in living."[3, p.9]

Most who attempted to interpret what they saw did so with good intentions. Their motivations were generally humanistic or religious.[3,4] "They wanted to tell an unsuspecting America about colonial holdings, pockets of poverty, cycles, syndromes, degradation, squalor, despair and hunger. There was much America needed to know, especially if it were to support a War on poverty and related progressiveness."[3, p.10]

As a result, an explosion of books, articles, documentaries, films and tapes appeared and changed Appalachia in the public's mind "from a place to a condition. Inadvertently . . . Apalachians were some extent dehumanized in this process . . . Many of our young denied their origins. Appalachia came to represent something awful in American life."[3, p.10]

However, a few of the writers who contributed to this explosion of information viewed Appalachia differently. Some of their works can be found amidst the poetry, novels, photographic essays, collections of folklore and music, and in the newspapers and journals of the region. Some of them are Appalachian natives.

These writers reported adversity, but in its midst they discovered a great richness in the human spirit. They discovered within Appalachian people an ability to find and appreciate beauty in simple things that are difficult to quantify.[3] They recognized a remarkable sense of humor. Traditions which were indicative of lives lived in harmony with nature were apparent. When examined closely, Appalachian people displayed highly developed skills in a variety of areas. They were remarkably self-sufficient, in spite of adverse conditions.[5]

Unemployment has been a chronic problem in Appalachia for many years. It has been recognized since at least the 1920's that many Appalachian people have migrated out of the southern mountains in search of better employment opportunities.[1,6,7] Most of these people have traditionally gone north into large industrial areas. By many accounts, the great majority remain homesick for the land, their families, and their former way of life. Many long for the day when they can return home.[6,7,8] Many of these individuals struggle to become "bicultural," adapting to the dominant American culture in the work place, yet retaining their own cultural values and customs at home.

This paper examines the values of the Appalachian people. It is recognized that this is but one aspect of the culture which occupational therapists need to understand. However, it is a critical component, as misperceptions in this area may contribute inadvertently to further disservice and dehumanization of the patients we treat.

The discussion of values is presented within an historical context so that the reader may understand how these values developed over time. The literature of this culture is rich in folklore, stories, tales and humorous expressions.[3,5,8,9,10] The author, a native of Appalachia, draws upon these to illustrate and clarify certain values. The intent is to present accurate, typical examples from the culture.

The content is applicable for therapists who may treat patients within Appalachia itself, and for those therapists who may encounter Appalachian natives who have left home. Both groups of patients will possess the values of their native culture, and these values will have an effect on the behaviors which therapists observe and treat. The following is a discussion of these values.

Religion. Most Appalachian values are rooted in religious sources. When the region was initially settled, centralized organization of churches was impractical and formally educated clergy were often unavailable. Thus, locally autonomous sects evolved in which the fundamentals of the Christian faith were stressed by community leaders.[10]

Appalachia has since been visited by many missionaries from "mainline denominations"[10, p.5] who often sought to save individuals from the influence of their local churches, which were viewed as a hindrance to social progress.[10] However, there has been a lack of recognition for the positive roles of comfort and support which these local churches have played in the lives of the people.

The basic belief system is based upon the premise that human beings are fallible. People know what should be done in various situations but often fail to do it. This is viewed as the ultimate human tragedy.[10] As one author notes, "it is not that our lives are more tragic than others; it is just that we more readily recognize them as being so."[11, p.29] In addition, loneliness is accepted as a natural part of the human condition. These concepts of loneliness and personal tragedy add a different perspective to the basic independence that Appalachian people are noted for.[11]

As a balance for these feelings of loneliness and failure, human beings are loved and "saved" by Christ, and this is the "good news" which is celebrated. People do not expect rewards in this life, but look forward to another life, and unpleasant conditions or disappointments in this life are thus accepted within the overall continuum of life on earth and the life hereafter.[10]

Individualism, Self-Reliance and Pride. These characteristics have been most often associated with Appalachian mountain people. Initially, they were necessary for survival. The original settlers of the region were anti-establishment revolutionaries seeking freedom. Many fought in the Revolutionary War to gain their freedom. Aware of their own struggles, they were also sensitive to the rights of others. They took care, as well, to ensure that their own individual pursuits did not endanger the rights of anyone else.[11] From this heritage has grown a long held skepticism of authority and of strangers claiming to bear good news. Considering the history of continued exploitation in the region, this current skepticism is understandable.

Belief in independence and self-reliance is still strong today, regardless of whether or not it is truly attainable.[11] Individuals prefer to do things for themselves, even if impractical. There is satisfaction in making one's clothes or furniture, building a house, growing your own vegetables, repairing an automobile. There is a sense of pride in this type of self-reliance.[10]

There is also a sense of adventure in testing one's abilities in a variety of situations. As one native of the region has written:

> I could have gotten along without some of my adventures, but they are important to me, because they put me in touch with other persons and skills. I feel good about being able to do a little of a lot of things, and if it became necessary, I could probably make a living at one or the other skills. The point though is not that what I can do in one or the other of these areas is important as an end. It's what it does inside me that is

important. I am not just what my title or credentials say I am. I am a lot of other things.[11, p.32]

Mountain people also do not want to be "beholden to other people."[10, p.510] Individuals often do not like to ask for help, preferring instead to struggle alone, even when in great need. The value of self-reliance may be stronger than the desire to ask for help in certain situations.

Appalachian people continue to cherish solitude.[10,11] Time spent in quiet reflection is highly valued, whether or not one can find a separate place to be alone. It is during these periods of reflection that people sort out the events of their lives and integrate them into the whole of their existence.

Neighborliness and Hospitality. Appalachian people have always been quick to offer assistance to one another. Neighborliness and hospitality, once critical for survival, remain among the traditions of the culture today.

Historically, even strangers stranded by a storm, or perhaps lost, would be offered assistance. To compliment a mountain family by calling them "clever" meant that they were very hospitable and generous with everything they gave to others, regardless of their own limited resources.[10] For example, a story has been told of a family who had only corn bread and sorghum (molasses) to eat. When a neighbor visited them he was told by the host, "Just reach and get anything you want."[10, p.510]

This value is now more often reflected by extending an invitation for supper to an afternoon visitor, or perhaps inviting an evening guest to stay the night. These spontaneous offers are genuine and very different from much of the rest of the country today, where more formal arrangements made well in advance are the norm.[10]

In addition, one is likely to be given a gift upon departing a home, such as canned goods, freshly squeezed cider, vegetables, or a homemade cake. This is not unusual even after a brief visit.[12]

Familism. Appalachian people have been described as family oriented and deeply loyal, even to extended family members— aunts, uncles, cousins, in-laws. This loyalty has been observed by "outsiders" and sometimes viewed negatively as a sense of obligation or duty which prevents free choices. Those within the culture have acknowledged an obligation to family, but it has been underscored by a deep sense of genuine caring.[10,11,12] In addition, people have always had a sense of identity with a specific family group.[10]

It is not uncommon to find an Appalachian native, working in a northern city, absent from work in order to attend the funeral of a distant cousin. Given the consequences of losing a job because funeral leaves do not extend beyond the nuclear family, this person will attend the cousin's funeral. Supervisors in northern industries are often perplexed by such behavior in an otherwise responsible, productive employee.[10]

Appalachian families will also open their homes to relatives for extended periods of time. Social service agencies often perceive "overcrowding" and identify it as a problem when a family takes in many relatives until they can find jobs and places of their own to live. It is not, however, always defined as problematic or unusual to those involved.[10,12] Families gather during holidays in similar fashion. Many people may gather in one home, regardless of its size, for entire holiday periods. The pleasures of sharing stories and enjoying one another's company far outweigh the inconvenience of limited space.

Human Relationship. Personal relationships are valued extremely highly and friendships are counted among the treasures of Appalachian people. It is more important to get along well with others than it is to make conflicting true feelings known. Individuals sometimes agree to all sorts of group meetings or appointments, knowing they can not attend, rather than appearing impolite. This value of preserving personal relationships with one another, coupled with a tolerance of others' differences and pursuits, is one of the reasons that confrontation politics often fail in Appalachia.[10]

However, when individuals perceive a real threat to themselves or their families, they will take a stand, as did the Widow Combs, Jink Ray, and others when they stopped strip miners who came on their land.[10, p.512, 13] All individuals are judged on a personal basis, rather than on how they look or what their credentials or accomplishments are. Children are taught from very early ages that one person is as good as another, but no better, and that everyone is due basic rights and dignity.[10,11,12]

Love of Place. There is an abiding sense of attachment to the place where one was born, grew up, and lived. One never forgets this home place, and individuals who do leave home go back to visit as often as possible.[9,10,11] One of the first questions asked of any stranger is "Where are you from?" People are oriented around places. As a result, Appalachian people are rarely inclined to feel adrift, without a feeling for where they came from or who their people are.[11]

This attachment to one's place appears to be one of the central, unifying values of mountain people. Many folksongs reflect a deep regard for the land where one was born. This value poses a problem for young people today who are given the message, usually in school, that they should leave the mountains to find a "better" life.[4,10,14] Those from outside the culture often fail to understand this value and are generally perplexed by it.

Modesty. Because southern highlanders believe all people are equal, they do not feel that anyone should boast or "put on airs." People do not brag about their own virtues or achievements and there is little competition, except perhaps in sports. Accomplished musicians, craftsmen, or even politicians will often speak disparaging words about themselves and their abilities before proceeding to demonstrate a high level of skill in their chosen fields.[10] There is a strong sense of personal modesty.

Mountaineers tend to have a fairly realistic view of personal abilities, but they do not take themselves too seriously. Because of the belief that human beings may fail, people do not become cynical or intolerant as those outside the culture may when someone does fail, or makes a mistake. No one is expected to be perfect. These beliefs make Appalachian people at peace with themselves. They do not pretend they are something they are not.[10]

Sense of Beauty. A sense of beauty pervades mountain life, and an appreciation of the beauty in nature is found in the literature and in the art forms of the culture. There are art forms, although some of these have been labeled "crude" by those outside the culture.[10] It is common to find many artistic expressions associated with exceptional craftsmanship in woodworking; in the pottery; in quilting; and in the spinning, dyeing, and weaving of materials. People have taken time to make household items attractive and to create a sense of beauty within even the most modest homes.[10]

There is also a rich musical heritage associated with this region. Beautiful ballads and folk songs dating back several centuries to England, Scotland, and Ireland have been preserved. Ancient English folktales have also been preserved and passed on orally, sometimes in several versions as they have become adapted to reflect the region.[10,15]

Appalachian people have also been described as the "masters of simile and metaphor."[10, p.514, 16] Speech patterns sparkle with colorful language of all kinds. The daily speech also reflects the strong oral tradition, sprinkled with a great deal of humor, indicating the way in which life is viewed. Examples of expressions include, "He'd cross hell on a rotten rail to get a drink of likker," or, "He looks like the hind wheels of hard times,"[10, p.514] or "I feel like forty miles of bad road."

The Appalachian person prefers to alter, adapt, and recombine old expressions with a freshness and creativity in order to communicate to others the events of his/her life. The result is a highly developed art of oral rhetoric and story telling.[15]

However, Appalachian people are aware that those outside the culture frequently view their speech as incorrect and inferior. As Appalachian scholar Dr. Cratis Williams noted, "nowhere in the English-speaking world have 13 million people been made to feel so ashamed of their speech."[16, p.108] For people who become convinced that their culture is inferior usually consider their language to be inferior, also.[15] As one elderly native said, his speech might not be the "bestest English," but he had no trouble saying what he meant.[15, p.488] This man did not feel his lack of formal education made him less of a person, however. As he put it, "Learning and good words may improve a man's knowings but it haint nary made a body a better Christian person."[15, p.488]

Humor. Although those outside the region often view Appalachian people as solemn, in reality they have a good sense of humor. It has sustained them throughout many hard times.

Their humor is actually a part of the belief system about the human condition. They laugh at themselves often, even though they may fail. As human beings attempt to achieve power over others and over nature, inevitably failing along the way, they are viewed humorously.[10] Pompous people are not taken seriously and others may play practical jokes on them. Historical accounts of the region include many awkward or embarrassing situations with which the people coped through their humor.[12]

Sometimes the humor is indicative of hard times. As an example, the story is told of a woman who went to the governor to ask for a pardon for her husband who was in the penitentiary. "What's he in for?" asked the governor. "For stealing a ham." "Is he a good man?" "No, governor, he'a a mean old man." "Is he a good worker?" "No, he won't hardly work at all." "Well, why would you want a man like that pardoned?'' ''Well, governor, we're out of ham.''[10, p.514]

Patriotism. Appalachians value the freedom their ancestors initially gained from the land, and they remain quick to defend their perceptions of threats to the freedom of any individual. Mountaineers have historically filled draft quotas with volunteers in all national conflicts, with the exception of the Vietnam war.[10]

Contrary to a common misperception, Appalachian people do vote in significant numbers[10] and are more likely to support a candidate on a personal basis rather than on party loyalty. Candidates who are believed to be honest and trustworthy tend to gain the confidence and support of the people.

Work and Play. One of the myths that has been perpetuated by the media in such forms as several comic strips and various movies and television shows is that Appalachian people are lazy. In actuality, hard work is a long standing value of the culture.[12] Historically, initial survival required a hardy people willing to work very hard. When the work was finished, adults and children joined together for stories, songs, and dancing.[12] Children were incorporated into both schemes of work and play at young ages and developed skills in both areas. A natural balance was achieved in these two areas.

More recent interviews with adults who choose to remain in the region, regardless of hardships, reveal a similar pattern. One relatively isolated and very self-sufficient woman stated:

> No, I don't go to town only just when I have to . . . don't get out o' here to church. We try to live right here every day . . . People that go to town life, they have to get a job. And then they say, 'Well, I don't feel like it, but I gotta go to work or lose my job, so I gotta go.' That's one thing wonderful to live out. If you wanta take off a hour or two, you can . . . If I wanta work all the time, I do. And if I don't want to, I don't.[17, p.46]

These people view modern man as having lost the technique of enjoying time for itself,[16] the art of ''sitting for a spell'' to visit with another person or to cherish a moment in solitude. An isolated self-sufficient lifestyle still requires hard work and offers few modern conveniences. However, those people in Appalachia who continue this lifestyle achieve a self-directed balance in their lives and establish their own individualized patterns of work, leisure, self-care, and rest. These values have an impact on behaviors therapists see.

IMPLICATIONS FOR OCCUPATIONAL THERAPISTS

Therapists are accustomed to assessing strengths and weaknesses of individuals in order to plan treatment. The following is an examination of Appalachian values in light of the effect they have on individuals from the culture and on the patient-therapist relationship. In addition, understanding these values may provide a useful perspective on a patient's true strengths.

The somewhat fatalistic religious attitudes may encourage a passive attitude toward problems.[10] If one determines this to be the case, it may be helpful to present a problem as a challenge to be overcome by appealing to an individual's desire for independence and self-reliance. Because of the skepticism of authority, it would be important for the occupational therapist to present himself/herself as an equal in approaching the patient's problems and to engage in an exchange of ideas with the patient regarding potential solutions. This approach offers much new and useful information to the therapist as well as to the patient.

It is important to remember the strong desire Appalachian people have to remain independent. Therefore, it would not be wise to approach someone as if you were there to offer help or assistance, as the implication is that the individual may become "beholden" to you if the assistance is accepted. It would be better to structure the situation so that the therapist could observe the patient attempt a task and then provide an alternative, if necessary, by saying, "What do you think about doing it this way?" This promotes the equal exchange of ideas.

Seeking Help

Because Appalachian people do not like to ask for help, individuals who need it may not request assistance from family or friends who would often be more than glad to provide it. However, the literature indicates that when people perceive a need and know what to do about it, they will extend themselves. The essay "Hermas"[18] provides an excellent example of a small community of people who managed to maintain an isolated, elderly man in his rural home, even after he became blind. Their unique adaptations allowed him to retain his independence for a long time, and when he eventually became very frail and was taken to a nursing home, neighbors continued to provide emotional support until his death. Therapists might consider this as a model and identify the informal sources of support already available to patients who need assistance in order to remain in their homes.

Hospitality is a highly valued tradition and the therapist who practices in home health may be given an invitation to stay in a home for a meal or offered a small gift upon departure. However the therapist decides to respond, it is critical to realize that these offers are genuine. One must recognize that a failure to interact with people on this level could be viewed as an insult and have a detrimental effect on therapist-patient rapport.

Hospitalization Issues

The strong ties among Appalachian families are often reflected in the presence of relatives in acute care hospitals when a single family member is ill or injured. It is common to find several family members in the hospital 24 hours per day. They may take turns sitting individually in the patient's room, while the remaining relatives stay close by, usually clustered in the hallways. Hospital staff often complain of this as a nuisance and tend to disregard these families, as if they were only in the way.

It is important to realize that this pattern of behavior occurred within homes, before hospitals became accessible, and that the patient and his immediate family may receive emotional support from this network of relatives. Looking for alternatives within the hospital structure, such as family lounges on each floor, would be beneficial. In addition, this might be an ideal time to begin family education regarding the future prognosis and care of the patient, especially if the person has had a stroke or another condition which will require rehabilitation and/or some form of long term care. Giving family members small amounts of information over time and allowing questions to be answered as they arise might be more successful than waiting until discharge and overloading the family with too much information at once.

Because human relationships are highly valued and Appalachian individuals tend to refrain from making conflicting views known, a patient may indicate acceptance of a home program or a follow-up appointment and later fail to follow through. It is important that patients understand why certain activities are prescribed and that these activities are incorporated into the patient's cultural values. They will not be meaningful to the patient otherwise.

Patients may not return for follow-up appointments for a variety of reasons. If they have been offended, they are not likely to indicate it directly. Therapists will have to demonstrate genuine acceptance of their patients in order to draw them out during conversations or interviews and determine indirectly their true feelings. Therapists must be aware that cultural skepticism toward strangers may apply to them until their patients have had an opportunity to judge their motives.

Acceptance of "Outsiders"

One of the long held myths about Appalachian people is that they will not accept any strangers into their midst, leading people to conclude that health care workers from outside the region would never be acceptable within the region itself. However, the dramatic success of the Frontier Nursing Service founded in the 1920's clearly dispels this notion. Established to provide health care services to the people in isolated counties in eastern Kentucky, the Frontier Nursing Service founded regional clinics and operated a network of outposts from each clinic. Nurses originally traveled on horseback into areas without roads or electricity, and delivered comprehensive health care services. They provided pre-natal care, midwife services, post-natal care, assessed each member of the family who needed attention during home visits, and taught health and hygiene practices within the home. They went to the community schools and provided innoculations for the childhood diseases. Their years of careful documentation reveal an amazing record of success, with a mother-infant mortality rate below the national average. They continue to operate today, using jeeps for access to their patients.[19]

This model of health care delivery indicates that when services are needed by Appalachian people, they are accepted if the providers deliver those services without attempting to change the patient's basic cultural values. In sharp contrast to this success stands the model of public education in Appalachia, which has been a dismal failure.[4,14,20] Educators, initially from outside the region, insisted that children give up their cultural traditions in order to become more like mainstream Americans and "better themselves".[4,14,20] The result has been a drop out rate far exceeding the national average.[4]

The Role of the Change Agent

As change agents, occupational therapists must carefully examine what they are asking of their patients. This will require careful observation and assessment within the cultural context of the patient. We do not want to practice as other "change agents" in this region so often have, by pressuring our patients to adopt changes which require that they give up behaviors which have meaning for them in order to adopt a set of new behaviors unrelated to their own values.[4] Many of the social programs in this region during the days of the "War on Poverty" required that people give up a part of themselves in exchange for whatever services were offered. Those identified as "failures" in these programs were generally the individuals who held steadfastly to their own values.[4] Meanwhile, the change agents generally became frustrated and departed the region.

The love of place which pervades Appalachia should be recognized, particularly by therapists treating patients who are living outside Appalachia. This will require that therapists conduct careful patient histories in order to determine if a patient in Cincinnati, Pittsburgh, or Detroit, for example, really considers "home" to be somewhere in the Southern Highlands. If so, then one might expect to encounter homesickness, or a sadness, perhaps even depression.[7] The patient may also express a need for solitude.

This should be viewed within the cultural context of the individual and not as a separate "pathology" to be treated with traditional approaches. A community support group of similar "displaced persons" might be a helpful alternative, in order to allow people the opportunity to swap stories of home or enjoy their food and music together.

Because of the uniqueness of some of the oral expressions in Appalachia, therapists unfamiliar with the speech patterns may not understand some of the things their patients say to them. For example, the person who says "I've fell off a lot lately" means he/she has lost weight recently. If a therapist fails to understand such an expression, the individual will probably gladly explain it, if asked to do so. It is important to have the correct meaning, rather than guessing at it and subsequently assuming incorrectly, for instance, that the person has had several falls.

When patients become comfortable with a therapist, he/she is likely to hear their humor reflected in their speech. Humor is often expressed in the understatement. A patient may understate a problem, especially if humor is used as a part of a coping mechanism. Thus, the need for careful observation of the patient's actual abilities is again highlighted.

The Importance of Work

Therapists need to realize that work is highly valued within this culture. A person may have many skills but fail to identify all of them in an interview situation because of personal modesty. An individual might have a range of work skills in farming, chair making, home repair, auto repair, canning vegetables, gathering honey, and hunting but still respond only that he/she is an unemployed coal miner or textile worker, or that "I've just done a little of everything over the years." A broad range of skills could be seen as an advantage in a rehabilitation situation, as the person may already possess a skill which could be built upon if others have been lost due to a disability. The therapist must carefully assess a patient's interests, skills and hobbies and identify all skills.

Unemployment remains a critical problem in many parts of Appalachia today. Occupational therapists could assist people in developing employment alternatives by identifying the skills they possess and seeking solutions based upon these skills. Craft cooperatives already exist in some communities. Farming, woodworking, quilting, gardening, toy and craft production are some examples of potential income sources with the development of proper marketing strategies. Occupational therapists could expand their roles into this area and serve as useful facilitators, thus having an effect on the health of individuals in an entire community.

There are many other implications for treatment which are pertinent for the occupational therapist. The therapist who wishes to learn more about the culture will find a wealth of information in the literature. The references provided with this paper offer a good starting point for individual exploration.

SUMMARY

Appalachia represents a distinct geographic region within the United States containing a unique subculture. In this paper, the author, a native of Appalachia, presents information on Appalachian values. These values are explored because they underly the behavior of patients from Appalachia whom therapists treat.

In the second section of the paper, the author draws implications for culturally appropriate treatment based upon the values of the Appalachian people. Examples are given to illustrate value laden behaviors which therapists may observe and suggestions are made for appropriate therapeutic responses.

The future of Appalachia is uncertain at this time. However, as Appalachian native and scholar Jim Wayne Miller has observed, the future may be bright if Appalachian people can gain an appreciation for what is good about Appalachia—its institutions and values.[20] Occupational therapists may play an important role in this future if they understand and support the values of their patients through culturally appropriate treatment.

REFERENCES

1. Williams C: "Who are the Southern Mountaineers?" in *Voices from the Hills,* Higgs and Manning, (eds) New York: Frederick Ungar Publishing Co., 1975

2. Caudill H: "Preface" in *Voices from the Hills,* Higgs and Manning, (eds) New York: Frederick Ungar Publishing Co., 1975

3. Jones L: "Foreword" in " . . . *a right good people'',* H. Warren, Boone, NC: The Appalachian Consortium Press, 1974

4. Best B: "To See Ourselves." *Mountain Review,* 5:1–6, October, 1979.

5. Wigginton E (ed): *The Foxfire Book,* Garden City, New York: Anchor Press/ Doubleday, 1972

6. Jones L: "A Remembrance." in *Appalachia: A Self-Portrait,* W. Ewald, (ed) Frankfort, KY: Gnomon Press for Appalshop, Inc, Whitesburg, KY, 1979

7. Arnow H: *The Doll Maker,* New York: Macmillan Publishing Co., 1954

8. Defoe M: "Appalachian Poetry: An Introduction." in *The Uneven Ground,* R. Thomas (ed) Berea, Kentucky: Kentucke Imprints, 1985

9. Miller JW: *The Mountains Have Come Closer,* Boone, NC: The Appalachian Consortium Press, 1980

10. Jones L: "Appalachian Values." in *Voices from the Hills,* Higgs and Manning, (eds) New York: Frederick Ungar Publishing Co., 1975

11. Jones L: "Appalachian Values" in *The Uneven Ground,* R. Thomas, (ed) Berea, Kentucky: Kentucke Imprints, 1985

12. Sloan VM: *What My Heart Wants to Tell,* New York: Harper and Row, Perennial Library, 1979

13. Miller JW: *The More Things Change, The More They Stay the Same,* Frankfort, KY: Whipporwill Press, 1971

14. Best B: "Historical Overview." in *Uneven Ground*, R. Thomas, (ed) Berea, Kentucky: Kentucke Imprints, 1985

15. Reese JR: "The Myth of the Southern Appalachian Dialect as a Mirror of the Mountaineer." in *Voices from the Hills*, Higgs and Manning, (eds) New York: Frederick Ungar Publishing Co., 1975

16. Williams C: "Afterword" in " . . . *a right good people"*, H. Warren, author, Boone, NC: Appalachian Consortium Press, 1974

17. Warren H: "The Winds of Change Murmur Up the Little Laurel." in " . . . *a right good people"* Boone, NC: Appalachian Consortium Press, 1974

18. Best B: "Hermas." in *The Uneven Ground*, R. Thomas, (ed) Berea, Kentucky: Kentucke Imprints, 1985

19. Breckinridge M: *Wide Neighborhoods: A Story of the Frontier Nursing Service*, Lexington, KY: The University Press of Kentucky, 1981

20. Miller JW: "A Mirror for Appalachia." in *Voices from the Hills*, Higgs and Manning, (eds) New York: Frederick Ungar Publishing Co., 1975

Implications of the Model
of Human Occupation
for Intervention
With Native Canadians

Nancy Wieringa, BSc(OT), OT(C)
MaryAnn McColl, MHSc, BSc, OT(C)

ABSTRACT. The following paper provides a theoretical framework for occupational therapy with Native Canadians. Traditional models of care have not been entirely satisfactory with this population, as they have failed to come to terms with cultural issues and to recognize cultural stereotyping.

Native culture is first explored, both from a traditional and a transitional standpoint, with a focus on issues which are of particular interest to occupational therapy, such as role performance, role learning, work patterns, and interpersonal patterns.

The Model of Human Occupation is then applied to dysfunction in this population, with particular emphasis on psychosocial dysfunction. Several basic principles in occupational therapy are examined with relation to Native culture. Finally, the various subsystems of the model, and their interpretation for this population are discussed.

Non-native medical professionals have encountered difficulties in providing psychiatric services to Canadian Natives because of the significant differences between their respective cultures.[1-3] Existing

Nancy Wieringa is staff therapist, Occupational Therapy Department, Lakehead Psychiatric Hospital, Thunder Bay, Ontario.

MaryAnn McColl is Assistant Professor, Division of Occupational Therapy, University of Toronto, Toronto, Ontario.

The authors wish to acknowledge the information and support provided by: Ann Kerr, Senior Occupational Therapist at Toronto General Hospital, and consultant to the Sioux Lookout Zone Hospital Mental Health Project; Sarah Kejick, Social Worker, Lakehead Psychiatric Hospital; Rob Canton, Student Native Community Worker, Confederation College, Thunder Bay, Ontario.

This paper appears jointly in *Sociocultural Implications in Treatment Planning in Occupational Therapy* (The Haworth Press, 1987) and in *Occupational Therapy in Health Care*, Volume 4, Number 1 (Spring 1987).

models of Western psychiatric intervention have been found lacking and have been modified to more effectively meet the needs of the Native client.[2,4,5] One of the conceptual models used in occupational therapy is Human Occupation, developed by Kielhofner.[6-9] Although the model is " . . . based on generally accepted realities or requirements of Western life,"[7] it acknowledges cultural influences at various levels in the development and enactment of competent occupational behaviour. This paper will describe the culture of Native Indians living on reserves in Northwestern Ontario, and will then examine the implications for the practise of psychosocial occupational therapy, within a Model of Human Occupation.

NATIVE CULTURE

The culture of the Cree and Ojibway Indians of Northwestern Ontario has been under Western influence since the first contacts with Europeans in the mid 18th century. The introduction of a money economy, the establishment of permanent residence on reservations, compulsory education in schools, and recent developments in communication and health services are a few examples of contact with majority society which have effected change in Native life. The nature and effects of these contacts and the historical and present character of the community varies from reserve to reserve.[4,10] A discussion of Native culture on Northwestern reserves is then, at best, a generalization; however, it can serve as a guide to understanding of Native peoples. The following section will discuss the traditional and present lifestyle of the Cree and Ojibway on Northern Ontario reserves.

Traditional Lifestyle

Traditionally, the Cree and Ojibway lived a subsistence lifestyle in which the extended family hunted and gathered as a unit. The infiltration of the fur-trade and the establishment of reserves did not alter their lifestyle significantly. Trapping began in late fall. Using the reserve as a base, the family unit moved to a customary location to trap, and established a temporary residence there. In December and April they returned to replenish their supplies and to sell their furs. From June to December, they reestablished themselves on the reserve, and worked on long-term projects, such as home and canoe repair. Social activities were an important part of life on these returns to the reserve.[11]

In this lifestyle, a seasonal rhythm of time use was predominant, time being bound up with the phenomena and processes of nature. Time was not conceptualized in terms of divisibility and measurement, but rather was perceived to be always present and continuous.[10,12] The Native experience of time was through activity necessitated by the pressures of a very harsh physical environment. This concept of time lacks the monetary value it has in Western culture as something which can be scheduled, saved or wasted. According to Nagler,[13] Native people performed tasks with little reference to the Western notion of time; time had no objective value to them. Patience was positively valued, as was the notion of readiness to act.[12] Flexibility and sensitivity to environmental changes were required, rather than adherence to an abstract notion of time.

In their subsistence lifestyle, work was given value according to its ability to satisfy a present need, rather than future security.[14] Occupational roles were traditionally defined in the context of the extended family unit.[11,15,16] The male assumed a leadership role, due to his expertise in hunting and trapping. As provider, protector and transmitter of his expertise to younger males, the man's role was essential to the survival of the community. The traditional female role entailed raising children, preparing food, making clothes and foot coverings and preparing the catch of the hunt.[15] Social rank was acquired through age, with the elderly being most respected, through inherited status[2] and through recognition from the community.[11,17]

Socialization of the young was the joint responsibility of all the adults in the community and was predominantly informal,[14] fostering flexibility and sensitivity to the nuances in the environment.[18] As children learned to walk and were perceived as able to assume more responsibilities, they were given chores to do. They were continually given opportunities to do the chores if not initially successful, but rarely punished.[22] Skills were taught by apprenticeship under a parent or older sibling. Within the peer group, behaviours which made one child appear superior to another were censured, as individual superiority undermined group cohesiveness.[19] The child learned to do things within the context of the group, encouraging minimal self-reliance[21] and autonomy from parents.[20] Adult roles were learned in the context of the peer group, through imitation of adult role models.[19] Grandparents in Indian culture had a central role in socialization through story-telling and relaying legends.[23]

Imagery is an important dimension of verbal communication in traditional Native language. Subtle changes in intonation are significant, as they alter the meaning of spoken words.[5] Non-verbal communication, through actions and gestures, is an important part of social intercourse. Verbal expression of emotion and affect is negatively valued.[10] For example, the Ojibway language does not have a translation for words such as "worry."[3] Verbal communication is generally used sparingly, and social intercourse is not to be hastened.[4,14] Communion could also be experienced in silence, and eye-contact is considered impolite, relating to its historical association with bewitching powers.[14]

Spiritual beliefs were a pervasive part of the traditional Native world view. Individuals were conceptualized as whole beings, interdependent with nature, the gods and other people.[24] Native culture strongly valued harmony with nature, and was extremely hesitant to interfere with its forces.[14] Overt hostility was negatively valued.[15] Instead, the Native learned to retreat in the face of conflict[14] and wait for the environment to provide a solution.[25]

Religious power was viewed as something which could be acquired through dreams and patriarchal inheritance. This power allowed the holder to anticipate future events, ward off evil and control the actions of others. Supernatural phenomena were also invoked to explain disease and death.[15] Thus pathology often carried moral or religious implications.[2] Traditionally, illness was dealt with by a shaman, who was perceived as having the power to identify the source of misfortune and prescribe medicine, rites or actions to restore health.[15] No distinction was made between psychiatric and physical illness. The healing process could last from a couple of hours to two full days, after which the shaman was paid according to his success.[2]

WESTERN INFLUENCES AND LIFESTYLE CHANGES

As previously mentioned, Natives living on reserves in Northwestern Ontario are not free from Western influence. A steady decline in available game,[5] mandatory school attendence,[16] and increasing reliance on casual work[21] have combined to promote change in Native culture.

Along with this change has come a change in roles and role performance. Authority in the workplace is given to those who have mastered English and have certified skills. These tend to be the young people, rather than the older males, who were formerly respected for their knowledge and expertise in traditional matters.[11] On the reserve, the elders still hold positions of authority and are given respect by the younger generations.[27]

Other than the change in authority ascribed to different roles, the nature of the male role has changed in many communities. The reliance on welfare and the lack of paid work[4,5,21] mean that males are no longer providers for the community. In some communities, the social organization has been disrupted with high rates of alcoholism and gas-sniffing, of marital breakdown and illegitimacy and of suicide and violence.[19,28] Additional social problems include long periods of boredom and inactivity due to reliance on seasonal work,[21] and an overall shortage of work and recreational activities.[4] Consequently roles differ significantly from communities in which the traditional social organization has not been disrupted.

Certain roles, such as student and worker, are not defined within the context of the Native community. As a result, roles that were traditionally enmeshed, such as father and provider, may now be separated temporally and spatially. However, the Indian continues to be seen as a whole person[29] with no distinction between work life and private life.[5]

Socialization is a focal point of cultural conflict for the Native people. The curriculum of non-Native schools does not prepare the child for reserve life,[16] and instead fills children with expectations for the future which are frustrated by lack of opportunity and irrelevance on the reserve. The materialistic, individualistic values of Western culture hold attraction for some. English, with its broader range of verbal expression, has come to be preferred by younger generations, while traditional non-verbal communication is devalued.[4,30] In addition, the educational process, with its emphasis on formal teaching and adherence to schedules, varies significantly from the Native child's cultural experience. In order to fit the educational process, the child needs to abandon the informal style of learning adaptive to reserve life,[12] and take on a more formal approach.

Spiritual values have changed to varying degrees. Some communities have strong fundamentalist Christian values,[4] whereas in other communities, Christian "good" powers have been added to the collection of traditional supernatural powers.[15] In general, the Natives still recognize one Manitou or god, who transcends denominational affiliations.[31] Bear[32] maintains that the spiritual dimension of life continues to be the foundation of Native culture. Evil spirits are still recognized, and are used to coerce and modify behaviour.[4]

Although, the shaman is still recognized and respected in treating illness, Western medical practices are also gaining recognition. A hospital in Sioux Lookout Zone, manned by white and indigenous workers, serves the people living on remote reserves. White nursing practitioners are stationed at outposts throughout Northern Ontario and fly in to other reserves. Many of the communities are served by non-professional indigenous health care workers, chosen by the band council for their skills in health care. These workers may enlist the services of white health care professionals when necessary.

IMPLICATIONS OF THE MODEL OF HUMAN OCCUPATION WITH NATIVE PEOPLE

According to Kleinman,[33] diagnostic categories are problematic in cross-cultural psychiatry, since they are profoundly influenced by cultural perceptions of what constitutes health. Although the Model of Human Occupation makes a conceptual distinction between disorder/dysfunction and diagnosis, it, too, is influenced to a certain extent by cultural biases. The model defines dysfunction as " . . . the inability to effectively accomplish daily tasks and to enact occupational roles."[34, p.31] As is evident from the previous discussion, tasks and roles in Native society differ from those of Western culture. What constitutes competent or effective performance of these tasks and roles also differs between cultures.[14,35,36] Even the inclusion of the adjective "daily" implies a cultural bias as to how activities are organized in time.

Since occupational therapy " . . . seeks to promote maximum competence in occupational performance"[34, p.30] the occupational therapist needs to be well informed about what is considered competent performance in the context of the individual's culture. Although the Model recognizes the need to adapt treatment to cultural parameters, this is a difficult task. Western therapists view the " . . . world through categories, concepts and labels that are products of their . . . culture."[26, p.34] Culture influences " . . . the judgemental aspect of perception—the attachment of meaning to these stimuli . . . ."[26, p.32] This "cultural handicap" is especially important when working with Native Canadians, who have communicated a strong desire to maintain their cultural heritage as distinct from that of majority Canadian society. In order to respect this, it is incumbent upon occupational therapists to become aware of their own cultural biases, and of how they can influence assessment and intervention.

The Model of Human Occupation is proposed as a flexible tool,[6] which is largely applicable to Native culture. The following discussion will include proposals as to how it can be used in occupational therapy to meet the perceived needs of the Native client, as well as some of its limitations. For discussion, the ideas are contained under the subsystems proposed by Kielhofner.[6] However, as he emphasizes, these subsystems do not act in isolation, but are interdependent. Many implications developed in one section then may also apply to others.

Assessment

The Model advocates that the client participate in the identification of his or her problems and in the setting of his or her own goals. This is advantageous to cultural psychiatric practice as it enhances the probability that the occupational therapy program will be relevant to the needs of the client. How this can be accomplished with the Native population, however, poses somewhat of a problem for the white therapist.

Assessments which rely on verbal communication, such as structured interviews or questionnaires, may not be appropriate for the Native client. Although many Natives are bilingual, some require the use of an interpreter. Also, the Native client may be hesitant to offer personal information, as social discourse and self disclosure are customarily not rushed, especially with a white stranger.[14]

Many of the abstract concepts of the Model of Human Occupation have little meaning to the Native client, making assessment through discussion difficult. Therapists are therefore obliged to rely heavily on their observation skills, and attempts to make inferences about intra-psychic processes, based on behaviour. For example, in Western culture, the therapist may be able to deduce a person's interests and values from a discussion about what he or she enjoys doing. However, with Native clients, this information must be obtained through observing him or her in an activity. Even then, Native lifestyle differs from Western culture enough that such inferences may not be accurate.

Western culture's emphasis on productive behaviour is not shared by Native culture. In Native culture, for example, it is normal to spend time with others in silence.[31] This would be considered inactivity by Western standards. Since time lacks the monetary value in Native culture which it has acquired in Western culture, it is not wasted in inactivity. The white therapist must therefore free him or herself from the idea of productivity and give recognition to the different degrees and sequences that meaningful activity can include. The Model emphasizes the inclusion of play, as well as work, as a form of output. Also, the less visible preparatory and contemplative aspects of activity should be recognized as legitimate.

The Native's experience will vary from individual to individual and from reserve to reserve, as well as with the cross-cultural variations.[31] The therapist therefore should be counselled against making assumptions about the client's past experience. For example, a Native living on a remote reserve may have little experience in planning a meal and little knowledge of nutrition, whereas many Canadians, through experience or the media, have more of an understanding of this. Assumptions about history and experience need to be checked out individually before judgement can be made or an activity program can be appropriately graded towards meeting a client's goals.

Finally, there may be a problem in attempting to involve the Native person in defining goals for treatment. Rogers[15] found that "native men were unable to predict their behaviour in a hypothetical situation . . . " and that they demonstrated little tendency to generalize. In addition, their orientation to the present, rather than to the future, may make collaborative treatment planning and identification of goals difficult.

Some of these problems with assessment may be overcome by involving indigenous health care workers at this stage. The white therapist's knowledge of opportunities to meet these goals in majority Canadian society may be useful in proposing solutions with which the Native client is not familiar. Such suggestions should be left open to veto by the Native client and community, in order to avoid ethnocentric solutions.

Treatment: Some Basic Principles

Open System Principles. According to the Model of Human Occupation, the human, as an open system, maintains him or herself and develops as a function of what he or she does.[37] This view of the human being seems to be shared by Native culture. The Native person conceptualizes her or himself as an open system, i.e., an interdependent whole with other people, nature and the gods.[24]

Adequate feedback is necessary for change in an open system. What constitutes adequate feedback may differ between Native and Western cultures. Verbal feedback will not be effective when a language barrier exists between the Native client and therapist or when the Native client has more respect for non-verbal communication. In addition, praise for endeavors is not customary in Native culture.[38] Several authors[14,26] warn against praise and paternalistic tendencies in cross-cultural therapy, as this communicates to the Native that he or she is too inferior to benefit from honest criticism. Feedback should be objective and precise to avoid cultural misunderstandings. Given the collection, non-competitive values of Native culture, feedback should not be given in reference to excellence as compared with another client. A more appropriate form of feedback could be created by the opportunity for comparison with a competent role model.

Environmental Management. According to the Model of Human Occupation, an individual will engage in certain activities because of their value in life situations. In order to encourage a client to engage in occupation, an environment should be created which is optimally arousing to the client. Collative property is one dimension of arousal in the environment relevant to cultural psychiatry.[18] This is the discrepancy between a person's past experience and his or her present perception of the environment. A slight discrepancy tends to facilitate exploration and can thus be used to advantage in occupational therapy. Too large a discrepancy is over-arousing and will lead to avoidance by the client.

The poor attendance in schools and the difficulty some Natives have in remaining in jobs isolated from the reserve are in part a reflection of how the disparity between the two cultural environments can lead to avoidance of the novel one. In view of the many differences between Western and Native culture, white therapists must be particularly careful not to create a therapeutic environment which is too discrepant from the Native's usual environment, and therefore, threatening and counter-therapeutic. The potential to create an environment meaningful and interesting to the Native client in Canadian hospitals is limited. The sterile, impersonal environment, with its schedules, white professionals, associations with illness and isolation from the community would likely be over-arousing to the Native client. A more therapeutic environment would be found in the client's community, where the disparity between the client's past experiences and the present therapy environment would not be as great.

The Model's adaptability to cultural psychiatric practise is enhanced by its recognition of the significant role which the environment plays in occupational performance. In cultural psychiatric practise, it is especially important that the environmental context is recognized, since failing to do that can lead to misunderstandings and mistrust.[12] The Native client, who values harmony with the environment and posesses acute observation skills, may especially find these inconsistencies disconcerting.

The Native client's perception of the environment may differ from that of his or her Western counterpart. To objectively assess and create an environment which communicates consistent expectations for performance, collaboration with a Native consultant may be used to critique existing environments and explore ways in which the therapy process could be centered in environments more familiar to the Native client.

Group vs. Individual Treatment. A significant value in Native culture is community reciprocity. This contrasts to the more individualistic orientation of personal achievement which is valued in Western society. To capitalize on this value, the therapist should provide opportunities for Native clients to work in task-oriented groups in which the individual's activities contribute to group goals and foster interdependence and group affiliation. Tasks should promote cooperation rather than competition between group members. Wax[20] noted that Native children in the classroom would rather not participate than show themselves superior to their peers. When possible, the Native client should be given the opportunity to help other clients with tasks. The occupational therapy environment should be supportive. A personal rather than a professional approach will foster a sense of affiliation. The Native may feel discouraged about participating in activities which isolate or place him or her in competition with peers. Natives, who by necessity or decision will be interacting with Western society, may find its impersonal and individualistic attitudes discouraging. Native clients could be assisted to make contacts with people in the larger society and to develop friendships through demonstration of ways of interacting in Western society.

Teaching—Learning Styles. The opinion that some Natives have of classroom learning has already been mentioned. Because many Natives are accustomed to an informal style of learning and may also have a negative opinion of the formal learning they received in white schools, they may perceive didactic teaching or counselling as being irrelevant, compared to experiential learning. The opportunities provided for "doing" in occupational therapy, which are emphasized in the Model, easily adapt to this value. Before counselling is chosen for a particular client, the therapist should assess his or her symbolic abilities. For some Native clients, the use of experiential and descriptive explanations, rather than rational explanation with reference to abstract notions, may be more consistent with the client's experience of language and, hence, be more meaningful.

The three subsystems of the Model of Human Occupation will now be explored, with emphasis on implications for treatment in each area.

The Volitional Subsystem

The volitional subsystem is largely influenced by an individual's culture, as it consists of valued goals, interests and personal causation. It influences motivation and decision-making, including occupational choice.

Personal Causation. Personal causation addresses one's perception of oneself as an actor in the environment and of cause-effect relationships. Native child-rearing practises seem to promote the sense of personal causation by fostering the child's development of confidence in his or her own capacities. However, they also foster the sense of interdependence and collective responsibility. Certain activities and decisions are made collectively, so that feedback from the environment on personal efficacy is often not relevant. Several other factors also influence the Native's sense of personal causation. Native spiritual beliefs influence the perception of cause-effect relationships. Supernatural powers, through which one person can control another's action and health, influence the perception of the self as a cause of change. As well, the interdependence with the environment and the expectation that it will provide solutions effects that individual's ability to feel effective. In certain situations then, the Native, by virtue of culture, will seem to have an external sense of control and will not view activity as an appropriate nor effective way of dealing with certain situations at certain times.

The concept of personal causation is also relevant considering Native participation in white society. The lack of mutual understanding and lack of shared values could potentially cause a sense of powerlessness among the Indian minority. For example, the abstract systems and formalized laws of the Canadian government have no meaning for some Natives.[15,19] In addition, their economic dependence on the government and the mandatory but irrelevant education of their children could contribute to a sense of both ineffectiveness and hopelessness in interacting with white society.

Interests. The model proposes that underdeveloped interests or a narrow range of interests may be a reason for amotivation or inactivity. To restore occupational performance then, the individual needs to develop a variety of interests. In order that these interests lead to competent occupational performance, they need to be relevant to the individual's life situation. Because the occupational therapist may not be able to identify interests adaptive to living on a reservation, the Native health care worker or community member who understands this concept could provide this information and offer suggestions of how to actualize these interest in activity.

The opportunities for activity in Native communities differ from those of Canadian urban centres. Boredom has been identified as a problem,[16] and the provision of leisure activities on the reserve has only minimally resolved this problem. The therapist then is challenged to find activities which are meaningful and accessible to the Native client. When involving the client in activities which require special materials, the therapist must take into consideration some of the difficulties in obtaining supplies. Some reserves are accessible only by plane, so supplies need to be flown in. Budgeting and long term planning may also be necessary in obtaining supplies for some activities. Because these skills are not typical of Native lifestyle, certain abilities may have to be taught or may simply not be considered appropriate for the Native client.

In order to address these considerations, the therapist should investigate activities found by other Native people to be appropriate to their lifestyle. The therapeutic program may help the client explore interests and how they manifest themselves in both cultures.

In some cases, seemingly contradictory values may be able to be resolved. For example, team sports include both a competitive component between teams and a cooperative component among team members, and are part of the Native experience. Games from both cultures could be utilized to both assess interests already developed by the client and to provide opportunities to explore other ones.

Values Goals: Occupational Choice. Associated with the volitional subsystem is the concept of occupational choice. In addressing this area, the occupational therapist will be confronted with one of the most difficult issues among the Native population, particularly with regard to vocational roles. Vocational choice was not a traditional part of culture. Formerly, the individual learned to define himself with respect to others in the community rather than with respect to a vocational role.[20] Responsibilities were largely determined by division of labour, by sex and according to the community's recognition of an individual's expertise. At present, roles in Native culture are in transition, as already mentioned. Western influences, especially education, have widened the range of careers available to a Native individual, and many Natives do recognize the link between education and employment. However, the lack of opportunity for jobs on the reserves and the loss of traditional pursuits mean that the Native individual has to choose between career and community affiliation.[16,30] Native communities may not recognize education in Canadian society as a legitimate means to acquire occupational status.[17] The occupational therapist then is challenged to help match an individual's hierarchy of values with community expectations and with available positions. The therapist, with her knowledge of routes available in majority Canadian society, could collaborate with the client and other Natives to determine appropriate, recognized routes through which the client could gain occupational status and/or satisfying roles in the community. Again the therapist could investigate feasible compromises by talking to Natives in vocational counselling occupations or those who have found satisfying employment. Some Natives find seasonal employment an acceptable compromise between living off the reserve for a job and remaining on without.[16] Others take time off work in the fall to follow traditional pursuits. The area of occupational choice has many inherent limitations and will require much innovation, communication and negotiation between the therapist, the client, the Native community and the employer. Because work in Native culture was engaged in to meet a present need rather than to establish future gains, the therapist should ensure that the rewards of activity are consistent with the client's values and temporal orientation.

The Habituation Subsystem

Internalized Roles. Roles are positions in a social group which outline expectations for behaviour.[31] The literature reviewed gives few details about specific roles or role expectations in Native society. Roles are not temporally nor spatially distinct in traditional Native culture, as the community is both an extended family and a productive unit. Ambiguity around role boundaries is enhanced by the informal transmission of training for certain roles. However, role categories and expectations for performance within them, while different and perhaps less recognized by Native people themselves, may be useful for the occupational therapist in assessing Native clients. Before role categories can be used in assessment, the range available to the client, expectations for performance within each role, and the degree of flexibility allowed in each role should be thoroughly researched. This information would enable the therapist to identify specific skills required to assume certain positions in Native culture and, thus, to match the person's abilities to these role expectations. In both assessment and treatment the therapist should recognize the demands for role flexibility in Native culture.

Because the Native Canadian learns to define him or herself in the context of the community, role responsibilities will be in reference primarily to this social group. Although the building of permanent residences has divided the community somewhat, a household will still consist of an extended family, rather than a nuclear family. With the extended family as the context for many roles, expectations for those roles will be different than for those in Western society.

The transitional nature of the Native culture provides a challenge to occupational therapy in attempting to restore role behaviour. In some communities, family breakdown, alcoholism and illegitimacy, as well as the absence of traditional roles, are so common that children may not have role models which teach adaptive ways of interacting with the environment. The apparent conflict between aspirations of white society encouraged by white schools, television and magazines, and the actual opportunities and demands of reservation life create the potential for role conflict. Some Native individuals, then, will be caught up in the disorganizing effects of being in transition between two cultures. While interests and values have a more individual component and may have greater potential to be resolved by the Native client, the environmental limitations of this aspect of the habituation system cannot be as easily resolved. Occupational therapy should accommodate the need for exploration of various roles, as well as attempting to provide experiences with Native role models who have adapted to the discrepancies and changing expectations.

Habits. The development of habits depends heavily on the idea of time, and its ability to be organized into prescribed patterns. Temporal adaptation is one of the most central concepts of occupational therapy since " . . . the awareness or experience of time is a reality so fundamental that it influences and directs all action."[37, p.202] In occupational therapy, temporal adaptation is defined as " . . . the integration of an entire spectrum of activities, the organization of which supports health on an ongoing daily basis."[39, p.236] The concept of schedules based on a twenty-four clock has no objective value to Native culture, however. In order to identify dysfunction in this area and to facilitate the development of routines and habits adaptive to the Native client, the therapist should observe what is normative with respect to time use traditionally. Observations about Native time use, such as the details of their seasonal rhythm, need to be identified. This may be complicated by the fact that some Native people operate within both the Native and Western environments, and need to adapt to both temporal frameworks.

The therapist may have to modify her method of assessment of temporal dysfunction for the Native client if a temporal organization is not apparent. Since ultimately temporal adaptation must meet volitional and environmental demands to be functional,[37] and this process constitutes the base of a temporal framework for activity,[39] an assessment which evaluates whether habits are meeting these demands would be an effective way of addressing this dimension with the Native population. The approach to assessment, described by Barris et al.,[37] emphasizes present functioning, thus accommodating the present orientation of the Native client while concurrently establishing goals for change.

Implementing a treatment program to foster the development of a temporal framework for a Native client may be difficult. Since

Native people do not have the urgency to preform or the concept of wasting time, the schedules and daily routines which dominate our use of time need to be adapted. The therapist may encounter a client who is not ready to work on therapy goals at a given time. Although this is not considered functional in mainstream Canadian society, the concept of readiness is normative in Native culture and adaptive to living on the reserve. The therapy program, then, should allow for flexibility with respect to punctuality and initiating action.

The Performance Subsystem

Skills. The basic components of interaction with the environment are skills. The Model of Human Occupation emphasizes the need to teach skills relevant to the life-situation of the client. Different skills are required for living on the reserve than in Western society. The Western therapist, therefore, may not be familiar with the necessary skills or able to teach them to clients.

One area in which this limitation manifests itself, and which is a common concern in psychosocial dysfunction, is communication and social interaction skills. Non-verbal forms of communication, which have acquired meanings specific to Native culture, may not be recognized by the therapist. For example, eye contact is a sign of disrespect in Native culture, whereas it communicates interest in Western culture. Also the situations in which verbal communication are appropriate vary between cultures. Social gatherings among Natives do not necessarily include conversation, nor is it disrespectful not to acknowledge another's presence. Non-verbal expression of emotion may be preferred over verbal expression in Native culture.

Many skills in Native culture will be different from those of Western culture. In order to sequence tasks from simple to complex in skill training, the therapist must have an objective understanding of the order in which skills are acquired. This process of activity analysis is difficult when therapists have limited knowledge of the activity and its skill components.

CONCLUSION

The Model of Human Occupation has proven to be a flexible tool for addressing occupational performance among the Canadian Native population. Its adaptability is enhanced by its minimal reliance on culturally influenced psychiatric categories, by involvement of the client, by its use of the environment in the therapy process, and by its emphasis on activity rather than verbal communication for treatment. Further exploration of how the therapy process can accommodate the different components of Native culture and overcome Western biases is required, particularly with respect to the temporal orientation of Native culture, its spiritual values and its emphasis on the collective over the individuals. This theoretical exploration can be complemented by direct observation of and interaction with Native people on the reserve, thus yielding more specific information about the practical applicability of these principles. Collaboration with experts on Native culture and testing of the ideas proposed will help to overcome the limitations imposed by Western cultural influences and lack of experience with Native people. The complement of theory and practise should contribute to a more comprehensive understanding of how and to what extent the Model of Human Occupation can be applied to Native culture.

REFERENCES

1. Department of Psychiatry, University of Toronto: Providing psychiatric care and consultation in remote Indian villages. *Hospital and Community Psychiatry* 29: 678–680, 1978

2. Jilek-Aall L: The Western psychiatrist and his non-Western clientelle: Transcultural experiences of relevance to psychotherapy with Canadian Indian patients. *Canadian Psychiatric Association Journal* 21: 353–359, 1976

3. Levine SV, Eastwood MR, and Rae-Grant Q: Psychiatric service to Northern Indians. *Canadian Psychiatric Association Journal* 19: 343–349, 1974

4. Armstrong H and Patterson P: Seizures in Canadian Indian children. *Canadian Psychiatric Association Journal* 20: 242–254 1975

5. Timpson JB: Indian mental health: Changes in the delivery of care in Northwestern Ontario. *Canadian Journal of Psychiatry* 29: 234–240, 1985

6. Kielhofner G, Burke J: A model of human occupation, Part 1. Structure and content. *American Journal of Occupational Therapy* 34: 572–581, 1980a

7. Kielhofner G: A model of human occupation, Part 2. Ontogenesis from the persepective of temporal adaptation. *American Journal of Occupational Therapy* 34: 657–663, 1980b

8. Kielhofner G: A model of human occupation, Part 3. Benign and vicious cycles. *American Journal of Occupational Therapy* 34: 731–737, 1980c

9. Kielhofner G: A model of human occupation, Part 4. Assessment and intervention. *American Journal of Occupational Therapy* 34: 777–778, 1980d

10. Nohner B: Activities of Daily Living on a Fly-In Reserve. Unpublished data, 1983

11. Liebow E: *Report on a preliminary study of acculturation among the Cree Indians.* Washington, D.C.: The Catholic University of America, 1963

12. Kirkness VJ: Education of Indian and Metis. In *Indians without Tipis*, D.B. Sealey

and V.B. Kirkness (Eds.). Winnipeg, Manitoba: The Canadian Studies Foundation. 137–171, 1973a

13. Nagler M: *Natives Without a Home*. Don Mills, Ontario: Longman Canada Limited, 1975

14. Sealey DE and MacDonald N:. *The Health Care Professional in a Native Community: A Cross-cultural Study Guide*. Manitoba: University of Manitoba, Faculty of Medicine

15. Rogers ES: *The Round Lake Ojibway*. Toronto: Ontario Department of Lands and Forests, 1962

16. Turner DH and Wertman P: *The Structure and Social Relations in a Northern Algonkian Band*. Ottawa: National Museums of Canada, 1977

17. Marula MS: Cultural and ideological foundations. In *Pathway to Self Determination: Canadian Indians and the Canadian State*, L. Bear, M. Boldt and J.A. Long (Eds.). Toronto: University of Toronto Press, 1984

18. Barris R, Kielhofner G, Levine R and Neville A: Occupation as interaction with the environment. In *A Model of Human Occupation*, G. Kielhofner (Ed.). Baltimore: Williams and Wilkins, 1985

19. Johnston P: *Native Children and the Child Welfare System*. Ottawa: Canadian Council on Social Development, 1983

20. Wax ML: Social structure and child rearing practise of North American Indians. In *Nutrition, Growth and Development of North American Indian Children*, W.M. Moore, M.M. Silberberg and M.S. Read (Eds.). Washington, D.C.: U.S. Government Printing Office, 1969

21. Tanner A: Occupation and life style in two minority communities. In *Conflict in Culture: Problems of Developmental Change Among the Cree*, N.A. Chance (Ed.). Canadian Research for Anthropology, 1968

22. Sindell PS: Some discontinuities in the enculturation of Mistassini Cree children. In *Conflict in Culture: Problems of Developmental Change Among the Cree*, N.A. Chance (Ed.). Canadian Research for Anthropology, 1968

23. Higgins EG: *Whitefish Lake Ojibway Memories*. Cobalt, Ontario: Highway Bookshop, 1982

24. Albon J: American Indian relocation. In *Minority Reserves: Comparative Views of Reactions to Subordination*, M. Kurokawa. Philadelphia: Random House, 1970

25. Blue AW and Blue MA: The trail of stress. *The Canadian Journal of Nature Studies* 1: (2), 311–317, 1981

26. Samovar LA, Porter RE and Jain NC: *Understanding Intercultural Communication*. Belmont, California: Wadsworth Publishing Company, 1981

27. Pelz M, Merskey H, Brant C, Patterson PGR and Heseltine GFO: Clinical data from a psychiatric service to a group of native people. *Canadian Journal of Psychiatry* 26: 345–348, 1981

28. Department of Indian Affairs and North Development: *Indian Conditions: A Survey*. Ottawa: Author, 1980

29. Spence A: Indian culture. In *Indians Without Tipis*, D.B. Sealey and V.B. Kirkness (Eds.). Winnipeg, Manitoba: The Canadian Studies Foundation, 1973

30. Castellano MS: Vocation or identity: The dilemma of Indian youth in Waubageshing. *The Only Good Indian*. Toronto: New Press, 1974

31. Kirkness VJ: Integrating into an Indian-Metis community. In *Indians Without Tipis*, D.B. Sealey and V.J. Kirkness (Eds.). Winnipeg, Manitoba: The Canadian Studies Foundation, 1973b

32. Bear L: Introduction. In *Pathway to Self Determination: Canadian Indians and the Canadian State*, L. Bear, M. Boldt and J.A. Long. Toronto: University of Toronto Press, 1984

33. Kleinman A: Editorial: Major conceptual and research issues for cultural (anthropological) psychiatry. *Culture, Medicine and Psychiatry* 4: 3–13, 1980

34. Rogers JC: Order and disorder in medicine and occupational therapy. *American Journal of Occupational Therapy* 36: 29–35, 1982

35. Gallimore R, Boogs JW and Jordan C: *Cultural Behaviour and Education: A Study of Hawaiian Americans.* Beverly Hills, California: Sage Publications, Inc, 1974

36. Ogbu JU: Origins of human competence: A cultural-ecological perspective. *Child Development* 52: 413–429, 1981

37. Barris R, Kielhofner G and Hawkins Watts J: *Psychosocial Occupational Therapy: practise in a pluralistic arena.* Laurel, Maryland: RAMSCO Publishing Company, 1983

38. Wawatay News: Respect My Child, p.28. October, 1984

39. Kielhofner G: Temporal adaptation: a conceptual framework for occupational therapy. *The American Journal of Occupational Therapy* 31: 235–242, 1977

A Cross-Cultural Investigation
of Occupational Role

Michelle Iannone, MA, OTR

ABSTRACT. The occupational behavior approach has been proposed as a generic frame of reference for occupational therapy, yet is has not specifically addressed the influence of cultural variation on its theory base. This article critically investigates the concept of occupational role, one of its central concepts, from a cross-cultural point of view. The literature on role theory and on Hispanic and Anglo-American values is reviewed. A study which described the occupational role enactment of a physically disabled Colombian adolescent female using the life history method is then discussed in terms of the literature. Finally, cultural implications for theory development in this area are identified.

Throughout the history of occupational therapy, both biological and sociocultural perspectives of chronic illness and disability have been used to evaluate and treat patients.[1] The biological perspective, which is associated with the medical model, has emphasized the diagnosis and treatment of disease entities.[1] In contrast, the occupational behavior approach, a sociocultural perspective developed for use in occupational therapy, has proposed a view of patients' dysfunction as a decreased ability to meet their needs and the needs of society due to the impairment of skills needed to enact their occupational roles. Although the medical model is useful for viewing disease processes, the occupational behavior approach

Michelle Iannone is an occupational therapist at Cedars-Sinai Medical Center in Los Angeles, CA.

The author wishes to thank Gelya Frank, PhD, Elizabeth Yerxa, EdD, and Florence Clark, PhD, for their assistance. This article is based on a thesis (*A Cross-Cultural Investigation of Occupational Role: Occupational Role Enactment Throughout the Life of a Physically Disabled Colombian Adolescent Female*), submitted in partial fulfillment of the Master of Arts Degree, University of Southern California.

This article appears jointly in *Sociocultural Implications in Treatment Planning in Occupational Therapy* (The Haworth Press, Inc., 1987) and in *Occupational Therapy in Health Care*, Volume 4, Number 1 (Spring 1987).

93

provides a broader view of the disabled person as a social being possessing life roles as well as a medical diagnosis.[2]

The concept of role was developed in sociology as a way of explaining the relationship between individual behavior and social order.[3] Role is defined as ''the behavior expected of the occupant of a given position''.[4, p.546] Roles, therefore, consist of *expectations,* or beliefs about what behavior is appropriate for a person, and *enactments,* or the actual behavior of a person in a given position.[4]

Cultural expectations define and shape roles. *Culture* may be defined as:

> The way of life of a group of people, the configuration of all the more or less stereotyped patterns of learned behavior that are handed down from one generation to the next through the means of language and imitation.[5, p.6]

By socializing the individual into culturally determined roles, society ensures that the individual's behavior will meet societal needs as well as individual needs.[3,6,7]

In order to understand the social dimension of disability, the occupational behavior approach has applied role theory to occupational therapy. When the proponents of occupational behavior adopted concepts from sociology, two decisions were made. First, it was accepted that roles are classified as sexual (male, female), familial (e.g., parent, sibling) and occupational (worker).[2,8,9,10] Second, it was decided that occupational roles were most relevant to occupational therapy and should be the focus of theory development. Occupational roles were defined as roles that had attributes that defined a person's position in society as well as the tasks he or she must do. With this definition, the sociological designation of occupational role as the worker role was expanded to include the roles of preschooler, student, volunteer, homemaker and retiree. Although it was acknowledged that sexual and familial roles may influence occupational roles, they were considered to be of secondary importance.[2,8,9,10]

In addition to these decisions, the following statements were developed:

1. Occupational roles are acquired in an orderly developmental sequence across the lifespan.[8,9]
2. Occupational roles enacted in childhood and adolescence provide the skills needed for adult occupational role enactment.[8,9]

3. Acquiring occupational roles involves a decision-making or choice process.[8,9]

4. By restricting physical, mental and social skills, disability can interrupt occupational role enactment and acquisition.[9]

Perhaps because it includes the sociocultural dimension in its view of disability, the occupational behavior approach has been proposed as a generic approach for occupational therapy. Yet, although it was accepted from sociology that culture is the shaper and definer of roles, the occupational behavior approach has not specifically addressed the influence of cultural variation on occupational roles. It has focused on concepts and values derived from mainstream, particularly middle-class, Anglo-American culture.

If a goal of occupational therapy, using this approach, is to assist disabled persons to reintegrate into society as functioning members, occupational therapists need to know what patients view as culturally meaningful roles in the community and how their culture views disability in relationship to these roles. What are the culture's role expectations for disabled persons? Are the theoretical decisions and statements proposed above accurate, useful and adequate for explaining the social adaptation of disabled persons from cultures outside mainstream American culture? The study that will be presented here was an attempt to critically investigate the concept of occupational role, as described by the occupational behavior approach, from a cross-cultural viewpoint. Because Hispanics comprise one of the largest and fastest growing groups in the United States,[11] Hispanic culture was chosen for this investigation. Before the study is described, a brief review of the literature comparing Hispanic and Anglo-American values will be given.

A COMPARISON OF TRADITIONAL HISPANIC AND ANGLO-AMERICAN VALUES

Although Hispanic culture shares characteristics in common with Anglo-American culture based on the Western tradition with its Judeo-Christian heritage, Hispanic culture is composed of unique characteristics which distinguish it from Anglo-American culture. These characteristics involve social stuctures and values which are related to this discussion of occupational roles.

Several authors have identified the family as the most important unit in Hispanic culture from the point of view of the Hispanic person.[12-16] For the Hispanic person, the family is usually at the "core of his thinking and behaviors and is the center from which his view of the rest of the world extends".[14, p.10] Furthermore, "a feeling of importance as a family member and interdependence are developed from an early age. Much of the individual's self-esteem is related to how he perceives and others perceive him carrying out his assigned family responsibilities".[14, p.13]

In general, traditional Hispanic family structure consists of the nuclear and the extended family. It is based on patrilineal lines in which the father/husband is the head of the household. The woman's traditional role of wife/mother is to nurture her husband and children.[14] Economic pressures, increased urbanization and exposure to other cultures, especially via the media, are gradually altering the roles available to women.[17]

While traditional Hispanic values stress commitment to hierarchically structured social groups such as the family, traditional Anglo-American values stress individualism, self-reliance and independence.[16,18,19] More emphasis is placed on meeting individual needs rather than group needs. Historically, interdependence has been more highly valued by Hispanic culture:

> In the culture of the Spanish-speaking people independence is not given nearly so high a value . . . people helped and were helped as the need arose, passing in and out of dependency relationships with each variation of their individual fortunes, and with no thought that a dependent status may be wrong or dangerous or undesirable.[16, p.133]

In addition, while Anglo-American values emphasize a work, "doing" and achieving orientation,[18] the Hispanic person may view work as necessary for survival but not something to be valued in itself.[14,20] Wealth and achievement are less likely to be criteria for success. Instead,

> it is through physical and mental well-being and through the ability to experience, in response to the environment, emotional feelings and to express them to one another . . . that one experiences the greatest rewards in life.[14, p.6]

Emphasis on familial needs and roles rather than individual ones and de-emphasis of independence and achievement all have implications for the occupational role concepts described earlier.

THE PROBLEM AND RESEARCH METHOD

The problem addressed by this study was the relationship between Hispanic culture, physical disability and occupational role as defined by the occupational behavior approach. To address this problem, the occupational role enactment throughout the life of a chronically ill, physically disabled Colombian adolescent female was described using the life history method. The specific diagnosis of the subject was dermatomyositis, a rheumatic disease with skin and muscle pathology resulting in cosmetic and functional limitations.[21] The subject had recently immigrated to the United States and was living in Los Angeles with family members.

The life history method is a qualitative research method which uses in-depth interviewing to reconstruct the events and subjective meaning of a person's life. It is a collaborative effort between the subject and the researcher. It provides contextual information dealing with the interaction of many interrelated variables over time and has been identified as a useful method for studying variables related to culture because it places the subject's experiences within their cultural context.[22] Although the life history method has not been used specifically for occupational therapy research prior to the study presented here, it has been used in the social sciences, particularly anthropology, to describe the adaptation of disabled persons over time.[23]

Although it is beyond the scope of this article to describe the life history method in detail, a brief description of how the method was used for this study will be given. Using in-depth interviews conducted with the subject and her family over a three month time period, the investigator attempted to construct a comprehensive account of the subject's life primarily from her viewpoint. The data were organized chronologically and were written into the life history, a narrative account of the subject's life from birth to the present. It included a description of events and how the subject viewed them. Using coding categories derived from the occupational role and Hispanic culture literature (e.g., student role, values, disease beliefs), the data were grouped and analyzed to answer research questions. The purpose was to identify areas for further theory development and to critically investigate some of the culturally-based assumptions underlying the occupational approach. The following findings are not meant to be generalized to Hispanics at large or to other cultures.

FINDINGS AND DISCUSSION

To fully understand the research findings and the person behind them, one needs to read the life history itself. A brief summary will be presented here. Liliana Rios (a pseudonym) is the ninth child in a family of eleven children. She was born in a small city in southern Colombia to a poor itinerant herbalist and his illiterate wife. At the age of four, Liliana began to manifest a variety of painful, disfiguring and functionally limiting signs and symptoms which continued into her adolescence. Some of these included open sores, swollen limbs, fevers, limping and the inability to raise her arms or use her hands for fine-motor tasks. The illness was treated by family members, folk healers and the professional medical sector, which eventually diagnosed the illness as dermatmyositis.

Because of her illness, Liliana was dependent on family members for self-care and other activities, failed school several times, did not graduate from high school, and had severely limited peer relationships outside the family circle. At the age of seventeen, after several years of effort, she obtained a visa to the United States where it was hoped she would receive better medical care. Liliana has had difficulty adjusting to life in the United States, especially to the emphasis placed on productivity, independence and efficiency which she calls "hard-hearted." She has had difficulty finding and keeping a job due to a lack of employable skills and the language barrier. She has, however, been able to find short term work (her first job) caring for children, a task she frequently performed for her own family in Colombia and one she feels she performs well.

Using the life history data, the researcher determined that the subject had enacted the roles of preschooler, student and worker. These roles appear to have been roles valued by the culture and the family, especially because Liliana's mother, who had little education, viewed education as a means to a better life for her children. Yet, because of her illness, Liliana was frequently absent from school and the family did not encourage her to attend. When she failed the school year several times as a result, the family excused her failure because of her illness. Liliana reported that she felt it was not fair for the family to have different standards for her than for the other children.

In addition, Liliana stated that she felt her family had overprotected her "out of love" and had prevented her from doing things for herself and exploring new experiences. For example, she was not allowed to participate in physical education classes or other games with peers. One family member reported that Liliana's brothers would frequently carry her on family outings rather than allowing her to walk. Her family bathed her, dressed her and fed her for several years, even though Liliana stated that she could have performed most of these tasks for herself. By overprotecting her, Liliana stated that the family prevented her from being a person "like everyone else."

In terms of Liliana's worker role, family members stated they believed that Liliana would have been dependent on the family for the rest of her life if she had remained in Colombia. She would not have worked, married or led a "normal" life by cultural standards. Liliana supported this view, stating that there were poor job opportunities and negative attitudes toward disabled persons in Colombia. Since coming to the United States, however, Liliana and her family's expectations have changed. Confronted with working disabled persons on television and in the community, plus increased job opportunities, expectations now include a worker role and a homemaker role in the future. Liliana stated:

> Now I think I can do anything. I hope to learn all kinds of things . . . I'm different than I was in Colombia . . . I feel more capable of doing things for myself . . . My family still comes first . . . The happiest times in my life were on my fifteenth birthday, when I did well in school and when I got my visa to come to the United States. The most important thing is to succeed. To be a free, independent woman. My own person. To have my own apartment, something of my own. I don't want to be dependent on anybody . . . Those are my wishes for the future. [24, p.176]

Despite this significant change in expectations, Liliana's occupational role enactment has been limited by actual physical limitations and by a lack of employable skills. Except for a factory assembly job which she lost after two weeks because of "inefficiency," the only jobs Liliana obtained involved child care and housekeeping. This has two implications. First, contrary to the theoretical statement that occupational role acquisition involves a choice process,[8,9] Liliana's acquisition of new occupational roles involved little, if any, decision-making on her part. Her preschooler and student roles were chosen for her by the culture. As for her worker role, Liliana's vocational choice was to be a veterinarian. Liliana and her family discarded this choice because of her physical, financial and educational limitations. She was essentially limited to whatever employment she could find.

A second implication of these findings is that, contrary to the statement that childhood occupational roles prepare for adult occupational roles,[8,9] Liliana was unable to find employment with the skills learned from her student role. This may be partly due to the poor enactment of the student role because of her illness. Instead, Liliana's sexual and familial roles, which required child care of younger family members and homemaking, provided her with skills that have enabled her to work.

In summary, it appears, therefore, that although the occupational behavior approach has focused on occupational roles, these roles may be better understood with further study of sexual and familial roles. Because of the high value placed on traditional familial and sexual roles by Hispanic culture, these roles may be especially important to the disabled Hispanic person and may influence his or her occupational role enactment. If unable to enact occupational roles because of physical limitations and/or cultural expectations, sexual and familial roles may be the only meaningful roles available to the disabled Hispanic person. In Liliana's case, role expectations were changed through role models (e.g., disabled persons who successfully enact a worker role), exposure to Anglo-American values (e.g., independence, self-reliance) and increased opportunities to enact adult occupational roles. In addition to these findings, it was found, in Liliana's case, that cultural, economic, physical and educational factors severely limited decision-making during the occupational role acquisition process.

CONCLUSION

The concept of occupational role provides a useful way of viewing social adaptation to disability. The findings of the study presented here, however, indicate that the theory base of the occupational behavior approach needs to be further developed to accommodate for cultural variation. Both qualitative and quantitative studies investigating the experiences of disabled persons from many cultures will be needed to meet this goal. It is hoped that this study will assist and inspire others to continue this work.

REFERENCES

1. Shannon P: The derailment of occupational therapy. *Am J Occup Ther* 31:229–234
2. Matsutsuyu J: Occupational behavior: A perspective on work and play. *Am J Occup Ther* 25:291–294
3. Turner R: Role: Sociological aspects. In *International Encyclopedia of the Social Sciences,* D Sills, Editor. New York: MacMillan and The Free Press, 1968, vol 13
4. Sarbin T: Role: Psychological aspects. In *International Encyclopedia of the Social Sciences,* D, Sills, Editor. New York: MacMillan and The Free Press, 1968, vol 13
5. Barnouw V: *Culture and Personality.* Homewood, IL: Dorsey Press, 1973
6. Hoebel E: *Anthropology: The Study of Man.* New York: McGraw-Hill Book Company, 1966
7. Ruddock R: *Roles and Relationships.* London: Routledge & Kegan Paul, 1969
8. Black M: The occupational career. *Am J Occup Ther* 30:225–228
9. Heard C: Occupational role acquisition: A perspective on the chronically disabled. *Am J Occup Ther* 31:243–247
10. Moorehead L: The occupational history. *Am J Occup Ther* 23:329–334
11. *1980 Census of Population, United States Summary.* Washington, DC: Federal Bureau of the Census, 1984
12. Baca JE: Some health beliefs of the Spanish speaking. In *Hispanic Culture and Health Care,* RA Martinez, Editor. Saint Louis, MO: The CV Mosby Company, 1978
13. Johnson CA: Nursing and Mexican-American folk medicine. In *Hispanic Culture and Health Care,* RA Martinez, Editor. Saint Louis, MO: The CV Mosby Company, 1978
14. Murillo N: The Mexican-American family. In *Hispanic Culture and Health Care,* RA Martinez, Editor. Saint Louis, MO: The CV Mosby Company, 1978
15. Rose L: *Disease Beliefs in Mexican-American Communities.* San Francisco: R & E Research Associates, 1978
16. Saunders L: *Cultural Difference and Medical Care.* New York: Russell Sage Foundation, 1954
17. *Area Handbook for Colombia,* 3rd ed. Washington, DC: US Government Printing Office, 1977
18. Weber M: *The Protestant Ethic and the Spirit of Capitalism.* New York: Charles Scribner's Sons, 1958
19. Zola JK: Social and cultural disincentives to independent living. *Arch Phys Med Rehab* 63:394–397
20. Sanchez V: Relevance of cultural values for occupational therapy programs. *Am J Occup Ther* 18:1–5
21. *The Merck Manual of Diagnosis and Therapy,* R Berkow, Editor. Rahway, NJ: Merck Sharp & Dohme Research Laboratories, 1982
22. Edgerton RB, Langness LL: *Methods and Styles in the Study of Culture.* San Francisco: Chandler & Sharp Publishers Inc, 1974
23. Frank G: Life history model of adaptation to disability: The case of the congenital amputee. *Soc Sci Med* 19:639–645
24. Iannone M: *A Cross-cultural Investigation of Occupational Role: Occupational Role Enactment throughout the Life of a Physically Disabled Colombian Adolescent Female,* unpublished thesis. University of Southern California, 1985

A Cultural Intervention Model for Developmentally Disabled Adults: An Expanded Role for Occupational Therapy

Arlene Morse, BS, OTR

ABSTRACT. This paper describes Chaverim, a non-traditional community based program, founded in the Jewish cultural context. Chaverim is a socialization and life-skill development program for Jewish adults with developmental disabilities. The program incorporates occupational therapy precepts of independent living, community integration, cultural identification and development of life roles. Specific details of program development and implementation will be included.

While this paper is concerned with service delivery in the area of developmental disabilities, recommendation for the applicability of the model for occupational therapy intervention with other cultural groups will be discussed. In this author's opinion, for a person with a disability to be adequately prepared to meet the challenges of full community integration, the meaning of culture in daily life must be understood and incorporated into life-skill training programs.

This is an account of how one occupational therapist developed an innovative program to meet the challenge of this task.

INTRODUCTION

Over the last two decades increased attention has been paid to the integration of developmentally disabled adults into mainstream

Arlene Morse is the Executive Director of Chaverim at Los Angeles Hillel Council. Chaverim means "friends" in Hebrew. This program was developed in response to the community assignment requirement of the Occupational Therapy degree program at University of Southern California.

The program has subsequently received the B'nai B'rith Hillel Foundation's William Haber Award and a commendation from the California State Senate.

The author wishes to express appreciation to Olivia Unger for her assistance in the preparation of this manuscript.

This article appears jointly in *Sociocultural Implications in Treatment Planning in Occupational Therapy* (The Haworth Press, 1987) and in *Occupational Therapy in Health Care,* Volume 4, Number 1 (Spring, 1987).

103

society.[1] Occupational therapists are recognizing the urgency to broaden service delivery into the community and to address barriers that prohibit the full integration into their community[2,3] of persons with disabilities. While great strides have been made to develop community based independent living skill programs, the actual training, most often, excludes consideration of the individual's ethnic, religious or cultural values.[4] Frequently, individuals leave these training programs with no further means for them to integrate into their respective communities. The young adults become discouraged by the absence of a meaningful context in which to apply their newly acquired skills.[1,5] The following is an overview of an occupational therapy program which has evolved over the last seven years in a non-traditional setting.

This paper describes the development of Chaverim (meaning friends in Hebrew), a community based occupational therapy program in West Los Angeles, California. The program is held in a non-traditional environment, Hillel which is a Jewish agency that provides social, cultural, religious and recreational activities for college students. Through participation in culturally based activities, individuals explore their cultural identities and participate as active members of the Jewish community while simultaneously developing socialization and independent living skills. The purpose of the program is to integrate Jewish adults with developmental disabilities into their cultural community.

CONCEPTUAL FRAMEWORK

Culture has a subtle yet persuasive influence on all of us.[6] The underlying principles and concepts upon which Chaverim was developed includes those of normalization, independent living, role development, and Jewish identity and culture. Culture is viewed as an organizing framework to guide behavior and give meaning to daily activities.[6,7,8] Within a cultural group, shared means of activities and values encompass a common understanding and cooperation with others.[6,7,8] Culture is the fabric—the rhyme, rules and reasons— which guides actions and behaviors that shape our lives.

The principle of normalization recognizes that successful community integration into life requires the acquisition of culturally normative behavior, and the need to create various culturally appropriate learning opportunities and environments.[9] The independent living movement has focused upon the social barriers to community integration and deems it necessary for people with disabilities to have the opportunity to participate in the joys and responsibilities of communal life.[10]

Within occupational therapy, the occupational behavior frame of reference recognizes the importance of individuals acquiring culturally and developmentally appropriate life roles.[11] The occupational role as discussed by Heard is the activity in an individual's life that contributes to society and thereby defines the person's societal worth.[12] Within Chaverim, the socialization process whereby skills and abilities are acquired, occurs in the context of Jewish culture. The subtle influences of culture on an individual's role within his family and community is incorporated into the therapeutic milieu.

Jewish culture is a blending of old tradition rich in customs and rituals. Concepts of self-reliance and self-care are interwoven with a commitment to community responsibility and the actual doing of actions to better oneself and mankind.[13,14,15] The temporal framework of the Jewish calendar is used as a natural organizing structure for Chaverim. Occupational therapists have demonstrated interest in incorporating temporal functioning as a useful conceptual base from which human adaptation can be better understood.[16] Vital skills for independent living are taught within this organizational framework.[17]

Festivals and holidays are celebrated not only for the transformation of ancient practices but to convey the contemporary beliefs of the people in the culture and community.[18] The Jewish life-cycle is explored to identify rites of passage such as Bar and Bat Mitzvah. Through participation in rites of passage,[19] a category of rituals that mark the passage of an individual through the life-cycle, symbolic meaning is defined within the practice of culture.

Significant rituals and customs such as Chanukat HaBayit (dedication of the house), where family and friends celebrate the establishment of a new home, help cement individuals' relationships with their culture and community. Inherent in Judaism is an adhering to an ideal for not only living a culturally rich life but finding specific guidelines for human conduct through the life-cycle, from birth to death.

PROGRAM DEVELOPMENT

In 1978, Hillel requested occupational therapy assistance to create a program that would meet the needs of Jewish adults with developmental disabilities and to integrate them into the overall agency's framework. At the same time, no occupational therapy model or assessments existed that incorporated cultural identity and community integration into programming. The initial tasks were to identify the Jewish developmentally disabled, existing resources within the public and private sector, and to design an intervention program for this cultural group. At the time of Chaverim's inception, there were no ongoing Jewish social and cultural activities in Los Angeles for the developmentally disabled.

Based on the principles and concepts previously described, as well as interviews with potential members, the goals of Chaverim that evolved are as follows:

1. To provide socialization opportunities for the developmentally disabled with their peer group—role models—the larger Jewish community.
2. To teach activities of daily living and life-skill development within a social and cultural context.
3. To enhance self-concept through development of cultural community role.
4. To provide opportunities for participation in the Jewish community.
5. To explore meaningful activity within a cultural context.
6. To coordinate a resource network of programs and services within the Jewish community at large.

POPULATION SERVED

The program begins the normalizing process by designating participants as members rather than patients. For many of these individuals, identification in the past has been based solely on the nature of their disability or disability peer group rather than a common cultural identity. Members are between the ages of 18 to 35 years old and are mildly developmentally disabled. Their disabilities include cerebral palsy, epilepsy, mental retardation and various neurological problems. Initially members were referred by word-of-mouth. Presently, referrals are made by social workers, other occupational therapists, Jewish educators and psychologists.

STAFFING

The functions of the executive director, who is an occupational therapist, include overall program, staff, fiscal and board administration. An additional occupational therapist is responsible for program development and implementation, supervision of a COTA and volunteers. Volunteers and other professionals teach art, drama, music and dance to enhance basic programs. Each year a new rabbinic intern is hired to provide Jewish content to the Chaverim program. The complete staff meet on a regular basis to coordinate activities. The staff serve as advocates for the creation of a resource network for the developmentally disabled in the greater Los Angeles community.

FUNDING

The initial funds for the Chaverim program came from within the Hillel budget. As the program evolved, a two year grant was obtained from a private foundation. Currently the Jewish Federation of Greater Los Angeles provides partial ongoing funding. An advisory board is responsible for developing additional financial resources. This board also serves as a community education network for Chaverim. Hillel continues to act as the sponsoring agency and providing in-kind support services.

INITIAL ASSESSMENT/RELEVANT INFORMATION

Once referred to the program, a participant is assessed through an initial evaluation covering the following areas: (1) level of function, (2) participation in cultural activities, and (3) time usage. Level of functioning is informally assessed to determine if members have the necessary social and cognitive skills to participate in programming (e.g., minimal versus moderate to severe disability). The program requires a minimum of basic socially acceptable behavior. A modified occupational history[20] is administered which includes questions on socio-cultural issues such as: Do you want to belong to a Jewish community center?; Do you belong to a synagogue?; Do you wish to belong?; Previous and present affiliation to the Jewish community; and, Future goals for participation in the cultural community. During the interview, a sample of a typical day is elicited to identify daily use of time and activities engaged in regularly. Additional assessments used when appropriate include the Matsutsuyu Interest Check List.[21]

SIGNIFICANT OTHERS

An essential component of the occupational therapy program is to work with families. With guidance families learn to be supportive of the member's accomplishments and identify ways to incorporate his/her new skills into the family life. An important goal of the program is to identify "benefactors,"[22] community people, who are trusted by persons with developmental disabilities to provide encouragement and assistance in everyday problem-solving. These persons may be Hillel or Chaverim staff members, students or others within the Jewish community.

A significant benefit of being housed at Hillel is the chance for Chaverim members to interact with college students in holiday celebrations and ongoing student programs such as weekly folk-dancing. Students provide age-appropriate modeling of behavior. A dual purpose is served as developmentally disabled adults are able to perceive themselves as a valid part of the community, and the community is gradually recognizing their status.

PROGRAM IMPLEMENTATION

In accordance with traditional occupational therapy's perspective of activities, the events of the Jewish calendar year are analyzed as tasks. Activities are assessed for opportunities of developing problem-solving and decision-making skills, activities of daily living, appropriate use of time and leisure, social skills and volunteer work. Members are assisted in identifying meaningful and purposeful activities that enhance their roles in the cultural community.[17]

Activities are held according to a weekly, monthly and yearly calendar. For example, Bar and Bat Mitzvah classes are held bi-weekly; holiday cooking classes are held in accordance with a particular holiday; and preparation for a yearly community event such as the Israel Walk Festival and Walk-a-Thon is coordinated with Hillel student activities and city-wide Jewish community events.

Planning meetings are held monthly to discuss calendar events, make committee appointments, and listen to speakers and socialize. Programs are conducted both on an individual and group basis.

Chaverim programs are divided into five major categories. Within each category are several types of activities and programs: (1) Holidays and Festivals—Activities of Daily Living, (2) Life-cycle Events—Rites of Passage, (3) Occupational Therapy Counseling, (4) Special Interest Groups, and (5) Community Volunteer Work. The following is a brief description of one example from each category of program. Outlined is the role of the occupational therapist and ways in which members participate in the program.

Holidays and Festivals-Activities of Daily Living: Chaverim members celebrate many of the Jewish holidays and festivals together. These major celebrations are utilized in programming for their life-skill development components, including activities of daily living, self-care and socialization. The occupational therapist conducts classes in basic holiday food preparation as well as works jointly with the rabbinic intern in teaching members about the actual holiday. Traditional festivals such as Chanukah (at which the familiar potato pancake is prepared) are opportunities for learning such skills as shopping, recipe reading, money management and how to work in a cooperative group. Similar skills are required for other holiday preparations enabling generalization of learning from one celebration to another. These holiday celebrations can be anticipated and repeated annually with old members serving as role models for new members.

Life-cycle Events—Rites of Passage: Bar and Bat Mitzvah is an important time developmentally in Jewish culture. In Judaism, the Bar and Bat Mitzvah ceremony is a symbolic rite of passage which traditionally occurs at age 13. It is the coming-of-age ritual climaxing in a symbolically-laden religious ceremony requiring responsibility in study and preparation. It also marks a developmental stage which symbolizes a person's entrance into adulthood with commitment and various role expectations that mark his/her social place.[13,15] For many Chaverim members, this natural and developmental milestone is perceived as being only for the intellectually gifted. Yet the very importance of this rite of passage for an adult with a developmental disability who goes through Bar/Bat Mitzvah can be especially significant, indicating that he/she has entered into adulthood.

A conjoint decision is made between the occupational therapist and the Chaverim member as to his/her readiness for participation in the Bar/Bat Mitzvah ceremony. Members have opportunities to watch peers go through the actual studying and preparation. A session is held where the occupational therapist delineates the responsibilities associated with preparation for the task. The commitment is further validated during a subsequent meeting that includes the rabbinic intern, where specific responsibilities such as attendance, means of participation and expectations are outlined. The role of the occupational therapist is to address problem situations that occasionally arise between the rabbinic intern, the member's family and the individual. For example, one member needed guidance in selecting an appropriate dress for the occasion.

Occupational Therapy Counseling. Occupational therapy counseling is available for members with problems in identifying interest, socialization, self-care and work. The occupational therapist assists the individual in seeking personal and program goals and guides the member in selecting appropriate activities. Chaverim staff collaborate and consult with other programs, agencies or professionals as needed. Confidentiality is maintained at all times and the member is always involved in the goal setting and discussion.

Often members and their families are unaware of available resources in the Jewish community and the occupational therapist helps in matching needs with services for this population. In turn, affiliated Jewish agencies have made a serious attempt to expand their service delivery, to include persons with developmental disabilities in community programming and expansion of vocational counseling.

Special Interest Groups. Small groups called Chavurah, gather weekly with the rabbinic intern for the purpose of Judaic study and informal socialization. The occupational therapist familiarizes members about social and leisure opportunities within the community, such as in synagogues and Jewish community centers, and teaches mobility training for participation in the various activities. In addition, the occupational therapist facilitates peer role modeling by post-Bar and Bat Mitzvah graduates for new students. Opportunities for peer problem-solving and moral support are available as members develop social and leisure skills.

Community Volunteer Work: Project Caring is a program for seniors sponsored by Jewish Family Service of Los Angeles. The program provides an opportunity for members to volunteer to make monthly visits to a senior citizens home. This participation enables them to develop essential skills for the volunteer role,[12] and be responsible contributors within their community. Members sign contracts of responsibility and hold several planning meetings for this activity. Workshops for members are offered to teach skills such as music, dance and holiday presentations to be used later with the seniors. Significantly, Jewish Family Service has twice honored Project Caring Chaverim members in their regular community awards ceremony, thereby cementing the integration process of these adults into the community.

SUMMARY

Chaverim is rooted in Jewish culture and utilizes holidays, community events, rituals and important celebrations which mark rites of passage, as an organizing framework for facilitating community integration for adults with developmental disabilities. Chaverim is an example of how one occupational therapist utilized professional occupational therapy training and traditional modes of therapy to develop an innovative approach to assisting individuals with developmental disabilities acquire skills for meaningful role functioning.

At present, program effectiveness is assessed through program evaluations from the staff, the occupational therapist's observations of choice of activities within Chaverim, feedback from members, and self report of member's participation in the broader Jewish community. While these assessments are important and play a key role in program evaluation and development, future research is needed in order to explore the influences of culture on community integration of disabled persons. It is this author's belief that if persons with developmental disabilities are to integrate successfully into their respective communities and proceed with living "quality lives," their cultural make-up must be valued and incorporated into occupational therapy.

Implications for Practice

The occupational therapists are among skilled professionals who can forge the link between an individual learning independent living skills and their application in the community. Therefore, occupational therapists need to pioneer, develop and implement community based programs founded on the principle of normalization. They also need to become skilled in obtaining support funds, developing resources and training personnel, as well as serving in an advisory capacity to agencies involved in developing community services and resources.

The following guidelines for community based occupational therapist intervention programs warrant consideration:

1. By teaching daily living skills within a cultural context, newly learned skills have applicability in the "real world." When community is viewed as what people do, and culture as how they attempt to do it,[23] the implications for practice extend beyond that of teaching isolated skills.
2. The individual's desire to be integrated with his/her cultural community must be taken as seriously as the obvious need for practical learning. Future work may include the development of a cultural interest check list to identify an individual's preference for activities that are of cultural interest and relevance, modeled after Matsutsuyu's Interest Check List.[21] Additionally, an instrument which task-analyzes activities and includes dimensions and symbols, rites of passage, rituals and customs such as Bar and Bat Mitzvah, etc., of a particular culture could be developed.
3. The differences between the occupational therapist and the members' socio-cultural backgrounds can inhibit development of the cultural arena as a valid environment for the application of practical skills.
4. The importance of using a cultural context to provide motivation can be misinterpreted by the occupational therapist for adults with developmental disabilities to mean their disabled peer group or socio-economic class rather than their ethnic or cultural group.
5. There are only general references to cultural issues in occupational therapy literature. This arena has not been effectively emphasized by writers. Consideration of cultural issues may

enable occupational therapists to analyze activities and include dimensions such as symbols, rites of passage, rituals and customs of a particular culture.

6. The education of the occupational therapist needs to emphasize the importance of the individual's cultural background to occupational therapy, particularly since wholistic philosophies are claimed by the profession.[24]

7. The tendency of the occupational therapist to gravitate toward the more secure and lucrative jobs in traditional and well established clinics and institutions often makes them unavailable to the population which needs them in a community setting.[25]

CONCLUSION

Concepts of culture (are) highly relevant to the deepest concerns and touch upon such intimate matters that they are often brushed aside at the very point where people begin to comprehend their implications.[6]

Chaverim, a non-traditional occupational therapy program for adults who have developmental disabilities is designed to incorporate culture as an integral component in developing the therapeutic milieu. The program is set within a community agency which was adapted to expand its current service delivery.

Unique to this program is the grouping of members on the basis of cultural identity rather than disability. The principles and concepts used in designing this innovative program are believed to be applicable to other culture groups and serves as an example of how occupational therapy can develop similar community based programs in non-traditional settings.

REFERENCES

1. Novak, AR, Heal, LW: *Integration of Developmentally Disabled Individuals into the Community*. Baltimore-London: Paul Brookes Publishing Co, 1980

2. Baum, C: Nationally Speaking Independent living a critical role in occupational therapy. *Am J Occ Ther* 34 (12), 1980

3. Tiara, ED: After treatment what? New roles for occupational therapists in the community. *Occ Ther Care* 2, 1, 1984

4. Lakin, K, Bruininks, H: *Strategies for Achieving Community Integration of Developmentally Disabled Citizens.* Baltimore-London: Paul Brookes Publishing Co, 1985

5. Programs for the Handicapped/Clearinghouse on the Handicapped. January/February, 1985, (1). Washington, D.C.: U.S. Department of Education

6. Hall, T: *Beyond Culture.* Garden City, New York: Anchor Press/Doubleday, 1976

7. Burke, J: Defining Occupation: Importing an Organizing Interdisciplinary Knowledge, in Kielhofner, G. (Ed.), *Health Through Occupation: Theory and Practice in Occupational Therapy.* Philadelphia: F.A. Davis Company, 1983

8. Geertz, C: Religion as a Cultural System, in Geertz, C. (Ed.), *The Interpretation of Cultures: Selected Essays.* New York: Basic Books Inc., 1973

9. Wolfensberger, W: A Brief Overview of the Principle of Normalization, *In Normalization, Social Integration and Community Services,* Eds. Flynn, R.J., Nitsch, K. Baltimore: University Park Press, 1980

10. Pflueger, S: *Independent Living.* Washington, D.C.: Institute for Research Utilization, 1977

11. Matsutsuyu, J: Occupational behavior, a perspective on work and play. *Am J Occ Ther* 25:291–294, 1971

12. Heard, C: Role acquisition: A perspective on the chronically disabled. *Am J Occ Ther* 31(4), 1977

13. Unterman, A: *Jews, Their Religious Beliefs and Practices.* Boston, London, Henley: Routledge and Kegan Paul, 1981

14. Donin, H: *To Raise a Jewish Child: A guide for Parents.* New York: Basic Books, Inc., 1977

15. Trepp, L: *The Complete Book of Jewish Observations: A Practical Manual for the Modern Jew.* New York: Behrman House, Inc./Summit Books, 1980

16. Kielhofner, G: Temporal adaptation: A conceptual framework for occupational therapy. *Am J Occ Ther* 31(4), 1977.

17. Morse, A: Cultural influences on community adaptation for developmentally disabled adults. AOTA Conference paper delivered in Kansas City, Missouri, 1984

18. Gaster, T: *Festivals of the Jewish New Year.* New York: William Morrow & Co., 1953

19. Myerhoff, B: Rites of Passage: Process and Paradox, in Turner, V. (Ed.), *Celebration and Studies in Festivity and Ritual.* Washington, D.C.: Smithsonian Institute Press, 1982

20. Moorhead, L: The occupational history. *Am J Occ Ther* 23: 329–332, 1969.

21. Matsutsuyu, J: The interest check list. *Am J Occ Ther* 23:319–322, 1969.

22. Edgerton, RB: *The Cloak of Competence.* Berkeley: University of California Press, 1967

23. Martin, D: The Guest Community: Asian Style Intergroup Relations. *Asian Scene,* (Ed.) Tai S. Kang, Special Studies Series, 78

24. Barris, R: Environmental interactions: An extension of the model of occupation. *Am J Occ Ther* 36(10), October 1982

25. Dasler, PJ: Deinstitutionalizing the occupational therapist, *Occ Ther H Care* 1:1, 1984

26. Hall, ER: *Silent Language.* Garden City, New York: Anchor Press/Doubleday, 1986

Cultural Implications
in Treatment
of Japanese American Patients

Jeri S. Kanemoto, MA, OTR

ABSTRACT. Therapists encounter patients from varying cultural backgrounds. The values of occupational therapy parallel that of the Anglo American culture, i.e., independence, self-initiation, and internal motivation. To be truly effective as therapists it is important to be cognizant of how values and cultural aspects influence interactions, treatment, and perceptions of ability and disability. The purpose of this paper is to explore some of the values in the Japanese American culture, particularly the second generation (generally 40–65 years of age). Values such as deference, dependence, hierarchy, duty and obligation, and external motivation are discussed along with treatment implications and recommendations for treatment.

Desirable therapeutic goals in occupational therapy most often reflect concepts such as independence, self-reliance, and self-initiated activity.[1,2,3] Such values are also those recognized as important in the Anglo American cultural set.[4] Recognition of the value system implicit in the therapeutic process is important, for it is possible that some of these concepts may conflict with those predominant in patients of other cultural subsets.

In patient-therapist relationships, therapists must be cognizant of the potential for beliefs to influence the way a person thinks, acts and behaves, and consequently, one's perceptions of illness and disability. In clinics today, therapists provide care for patients from

Jeri S. Kanemoto graduated from the University of Southern California. This paper is adapted from her master's thesis entitled, "Values of Physically Disabled Japanese American Nisei Men." She is currently the Education Coordinator of Occupational Therapy at Huntington Memorial Hospital, Pasadena, CA. Special acknowledgement is given to Dr. Ruth Zemke at USC for her assistance in preparation of the thesis.

This paper appears jointly in *Sociocultural Implications in Treatment Planning in Occupational Therapy* (The Haworth Press, Inc., 1987) and in *Occupational Therapy in Health Care*, Volume 4, Number 1 (Spring 1987).

many cultures. One such cultural set, which will be addressed in this paper, is that of the Japanese American (American born of Japanese descent).

The purpose of this paper is to describe the value system of the Japanese American and discuss how it fits with the theoretical framework of occupational therapy. The goal is to raise therapists' consciousness of how cultural beliefs can influence therapy goals and treatment.

Also to be included is a brief discussion of the findings from a study comparing the value orientations of Anglo American occupational therapists and physically disabled Japanese American second generation males. Thus, most of the discussion in this paper pertains to the second generation. The values presented are also prevalent in the third generation, but to a lesser degree. Conversely, they are generally present to a greater degree in the first generation.

To understand how the cultural background of the Japanese American patient compares with the concepts usually deemed important in occupational therapy, a description of each belief system will follow. The two values systems will then be compared and integrated. From this, implications for effective treatment will be developed and suggestions made for practical use in the clinic.

OCCUPATIONAL THERAPY VALUES

Achievement of goals vital to patient success in treatment are those most often reflected in the Anglo American culture. Constructs now considered important in the therapeutic process include "high achievement motivation," "maximal independence," "self-initiative behavior," and "internal motivation."[5,2] These are similar to traditional Anglo American beliefs profiling characteristics such as egalitarianism, independence, self-reliance, staunch individualism, and self-assertion.[4]

Motivation to achieve seems inherent in the therapeutic process. Reilly stated that, "our direct responsibility was for patient achievement. The achievement theme is our major frame of reference."[5, p.302] The therapeutic process encompasses use of purposeful activities by which the patient is an active participant toward achieving optimal independence and function. The therapist acts as a "catalyst" or "facilitator." Ultimate success is dependent on the intrinsic motivation of the patient.[1,5]

JAPANESE AMERICAN VALUES

Cultural values provide the backbone of behavior, actions and perceptions. It is the "generator" and judge of normal and abnormal behavior. Beliefs restrict and delimit how emotions are expressed and how attitudes are handled.[6] If true, therapists cannot ignore a patient's cultural values if they are to treat the "whole" person. Therapists must help the patient return to his lifestyle and culture, not their own.

Literature supports that despite acculturation processes, Japanese Americans still retain those traditional Japanese values brought to the United States by the first generation.[4,6,8,9] Discussion here primarily pertains to the second generation. It is this population most likely to be encountered in the clinic. However, it is important to realize that these beliefs are predominant in all generations. These values are present to a greater degree in the first generation, and to a lesser degree in the third generation.

Historically, emphasis in Japan was on the *samurai*-type family system. This involved a strict hierarchical, authoritative structure emphasizing duties and obligation, and deemphasizing individual rights and privileges. Great emphasis was placed on appearance to others and "saving face." The Japanese were also more self-effacing and passive in comparison to Americans, who were more self-assertive and aggressive.[10]

Dependence. Beyond childhood, dependence is often regarded as a sign of weakness in the Anglo American culture. Yet in the Japanese culture, there is a sense of dependence, or more accurately, interdependence that is fostered within the family and throughout life. This usually results in a less than autonomous ego, but nevertheless, is perfectly well accepted. Similarly, a child learns to maintain basic trusts in parents and other authority figures. There exists the implicit assumption that one will be taken care of should special needs arise.

Collectivity. As one represses personal goals for the goals of the group or family, it is evident that collectivity and harmony is important. To be "individualistic" is shamed and thought of as selfish. Outward conformability and thus emotional dependence on external reinforcement become important.

Duties and Obligations. Within a particular reference group, there are implicit expectations to fulfill. A child is taught never to forget about obligations to family and significant others. One's eventual independence and self-reliance in adulthood is achievable and respected, but only if manifested in accordance to the expectations of others and moral obligations towards others.

Hierarchy. The concept of hierarchy is the essence of all social interactions. The emphasis on vertical superior-inferior relationships is associated with achievement motivation and socialization practices that create a heightened sensitivity to the opinions of others. The Japanese language formalizes these distinctions by the many forms of addressing others depending on particular status within the hierarchical structure. Much respect and trust is placed on authority figures. Authority figures are not questioned.

Deference. At the expense of one's own individuation, deferent behavior to authority figures and significant others is evident. It is not uncommon for one to follow instructions and do what is expected rather than to question. An important concept is *enryo,* which is a restraining or holding back, deferring to others, or playing down. Seen from an American standard, the Japanese tend to lack verbal participation, especially in an integrated group, and tend to be inhibited in asking questions. They also tend to be more timid in the presence of superiors.[9] These qualities can be seen in the typical shy, reserved, stoic, compliant Japanese American patient.

Harmony. Saving face and preventing shame become important survival factors if one considers the heightened sensitivity to the opinion of others the Japanese person feels. Therefore, one may see unwillingness to admit, or hiding a less than optimal situation or event.

High Achievement. In both cultures, achievement is highly valued. However, it is valued within a situational context of fulfilling duties and obligations and expectations of others. Unlike the internal motivation that is the driving force toward achieving independence and self-reliance in the Anglo American culture, the Japanese culture seems to rely on and accept external motivating factors as positive influences toward success and achievement.

It is likely that although the Japanese American and Japanese value orientations differ from the Anglo American value system, the Japanese American culture seems to complement the Anglo American culture.[6] Both cultures are achievement oriented, although different values and reinforcements operate during the process. Because the two cultures complement each other, it is not unreasonable to speculate that therapists may unknowingly draw conclusions about their Japanese American patients based on their own belief systems when matters arise in the clinic that cannot be explained by any other means.

OCCUPATIONAL THERAPY VALUES AND JAPANESE AMERICAN VALUES

In a study comparing the responses of Anglo American occupational therapists (n = 20) and physically disabled second generation Japanese American males (n = 11) on two questionnaires regarding value statements and behavioral clinical situations, statistical differences (p < .01) were found between the two groups.[11] Patients and therapists were administered the Connor Contrasting Values Opinion Survey (CCVOS)[4] and the Patient-Therapist Interaction and Goals Survey (PTIGS).[11] The CCVOS was developed by an anthropologist to measure psychological and behavioral characteristics in three generations of Japanese Americans. It was selected for the study to assess the degree of retention of traditional Japanese values in a sample of physically disabled second generation males. The PTIGS was a survey developed by this author to assess similar values as in the CCVOS. However, these statements reflected behaviors and performance specific to a therapy setting. Results are summarized in Table 1.

In both assessments, patients or therapists were asked to rate, on a five point scale, the degree to which they agreed with the statements. The CCVOS included twenty statements;[*] the PTIGS included forty statements.[**] The widest difference in scores were related to hierarchy and duty/obligation values on both surveys. Other values compared included dependence, deference, and collectivity (refer to Tables 2 and 3).

Although results may not be conclusive because of small sample size, the study did suggest that values from the Japanese American culture may indeed differ from traditional occupational therapy values. Subsequently, it may be an important factor in understanding how therapy and the therapist relationship is perceived by the patient.

---

[*]Sample statement: You can usually tell what kind of a person an individual is if you know his family background.

[**]Sample statement. In general I am more likely to do something if I know someone else expects me to do it.

Table 1

Summary of Comparisons and Results

Comparison	Instrument	t-score	Level of significance
Nisei sample vs. Nisei norms	CCVOS	.80	NS
Nisei sample vs. Anglo American norms	CCVOS	5.10	.01[a]
Nisei sample vs. OTR sample	CCVOS	3.85	.01[b]
Nisei sample vs. OTR sample	CCVOS	5.50	.01[b]

[a] $t(19) = 2.539$, $p < .01$

[b] $t(29) = 2.462$, $p < .01$

Table 2

Mean CCVOS Scores for Each Value Category

Value Category	Nisei sample	OTR sample	Difference
Hierarchy	3.39	2.08	1.31
Duty/Obligation	3.59	2.56	1.03
Collectivity	3.74	3.00	0.74
Deference	3.16	2.44	0.72
Dependence	3.33	3.08	0.25

It also cannot be ignored that in the study some differences may have been attributed to female therapists being compared to male patients. Since this is a reality often encountered in the clinic however, it would be impractical to isolate it.

TREATMENT IMPLICATIONS

Although there will certainly be exceptions, one can formulate a picture of the typical Japanese American prototype. The typical Japanese American patient, influenced by the aforementioned set of values, can be characterized as quiet, compliant, stoic, polite, hardworking, and accommodating.

Compliant and Hardworking. There is an emphasis on vertical relationships and consequently on duties and obligations toward superior figures. From this perspective, the patient probably perceives the therapist to be a superior figure. The therapist is seen as the authority figure with respect to knowledge about disability and therapy techniques. The patient, out of deference to an authority figure, is compliant, may be intimidated, and is less inclined to doubt or question the therapist. To be otherwise would be considered disrespectful. The therapist, in contrast, perceives herself as the "catalyst" or "facilitator" of treatment and activities, not the "authority figure." [1] In such instances, it is the therapist who will need to initiate and probably persist in getting feedback, and asking for questions. The patient would probably feel very uncomfortable initiating the process. In addition, the patient may require some time in order to adjust to the role relationship discrepancy. With persistence and initiating the feedback communication, the therapist has a better chance of obtaining accurate verbal information.

Table 3

Mean PTIGS Scores for Each Value Cluster

Value Cluster	Nisei sample	OTR sample	Difference
Hierarchy/ Deference	3.40	2.06	1.34
Duty/ Obligation	3.61	2.50	1.11
Dependence/ Collectivity	3.09	2.49	0.60
Deference	3.11	2.72	0.39

Formal and Polite. Related to the hierarchical orientation of therapist-patient and the therapist perceived as "superior," the Japanese American patient may act in a very formal way and not feel as comfortable approaching the therapist with problems or questions. The patient views the therapist as "boss" and acts submissively. It will take a longer period of time for the patient to feel comfortable with the therapist. Therapists may need to make an extra effort to be empathetic in a non-threatening manner, and realize it may just take more time to achieve rapport with the patient.

Quiet and Stoic. In the quiet personality of the Japanese American patient, there is an emphasis on nonverbal communication. The therapist needs to be cognizant of this and be aware that it may be more difficult for such patients to verbalize thought. Therapists must be sensitive to this and may need to be more aware of the subtlety and implicitness in actions or behaviors. Again, therapists may need to ask for feedback more frequently, and at a more conscious level.

Accommodating. Compliant behavior does not necessarily indicate acceptance or agreement. Japanese American patients may sense a certain duty or obligation to cooperate because of external expectations that they should obey the therapist, since the therapist is there specifically for their benefit. Therapists, however, cannot assume that this polite, cooperative behavior necessarily means acceptance and total agreement with their treatment efforts. It is vital to develop a sense for the subtleties and make conscious efforts to initiate the feedback process.

Heightened Sensitivity to Shame. The Japanese American patient will be particularly embarrassed or shamed by failure because of a heightened sensitivity to the expectations of others and the opinions of others. He may be reluctant to engage in tasks thought to be too difficult, or activities at which success is questionable. Likewise, he may be reluctant to participate in activities perceived as childish, or in activities he should be able to do (according to the expectations of self and others), but cannot. Therapists need to be cognizant of this and respect the patient's feelings. The therapist's role is to carefully explain the rationale and offer the "just right" challenge. Thus, an element of success is incorporated into each activity. This is important in the treatment of all patients, but may be especially crucial in a Japanese American patient's acceptance of therapy.

Achievement. Very important for therapists to understand with Japanese American patients is the relationship between achievement, competition, and failure. Benedict[12] compared competition and feelings of shame and defeat among Japanese children. She found that there was an extreme sensitivity to competition and failure. She stressed the importance of recognizing that competition to the Japanese did not have the same degree of socially desirable effects as to Anglo Americans. Psychological tests showed that competition amongst Anglo Americans stimulated work and was viewed as positive. With Japanese children, however, performance decreased when competition was introduced and the need to perform was elevated. When the project became too competitive and thus more externally enforced, they became principally interested in the danger of defeat. She went on to state that the Japanese often avoided occasions in which failure might occur. Although this was not a study pertaining to Japanese Americans, its applicability is still relevant. This relates to the shame the Japanese American patient may feel with unsuccessful tasks. The patient senses failure in not being able to satisfy the expectations of significant others, particularly the therapist and/or family. The importance of others reflects an orientation toward collectivity. In addition, failure alters one's concept of oneself and therefore his relationships with others. Thus, one's particular status in a hierarchical structure, or family, can easily be threatened.

"Independence." The essence of occupational therapy is to eventually foster independence. Initially the therapeutic setting provides an environment in which the dependent patient can strive toward independence in a safe and guided manner. For the Japanese American patient, independence may not have the same meaning. There usually is a need for independence, but not at the expense of failure, shame or embarrassment. If the patient foresees potential failure or shame, the patient can fairly comfortably rely on the family to help with his needs, without these feelings. Thus striving for future independence may be more threatening than accepting dependence on the family.

To be considered as "disabled" or "unable," even if independent, may be perceived as more embarrassing or shameful than being dependent or protected (hidden) within the family. The family is thought to be the collective unit. There are duties and obligations expected within the family system that are not considered as being dependent actions to the Japanese American family network. Therefore, it is easy for the "disabled" family member to be taken under the wing of the family without feeling the need to be independent of them. It is more shameful, or embarrassing to have to rely on others outside of the family. Such actions would carry with it moral obligations, which that disabled person, in his own mind, would never be able to repay.[9,12]

CONCLUSION

Therapists need to try to understand the values guiding the behaviors that they observe in patients. When working with the Japanese American patient, the therapist may need to be the initiator in asking for feedback or questions. More time may be needed to develop a comfortable relationship and open communication. Finally, and very importantly, the therapist must develop a sense of intuitiveness and sensitivity to non-verbal communication. The Japanese American patient may tend not to be very verbal and a lot can be missed if the therapist is not sensitive to this. Therapists must recognize the importance of shame and significance of the expectations of others in their Japanese American patients. To ensure successful treatment, therapists need to offer appropriate tasks in an effort to minimize shame from lack of success.

If therapists are to be effective in their treatment, they must consider making suggestions and recommendations that are within the realm of the patient's own value system. Cultural aspects inherently influence one's values. The culture of the Japanese American patient is one that complements the Anglo American and occupational therapy culture. Yet, if one dissects it, it is found to be significantly different. To successfully treat the Japanese American patient, the therapist must recognize the importance of such values of hierarchy, collectivity, deference, duty/obligation, dependence, externally motivated achievement, shame, and a heightened sensitivity of the significance of others.

REFERENCES

1. Yerxa, E. 1966 Eleanor Clarke Slagle Lecture: Authentic occupational therapy. *Am J Occup Ther* 21(1): 1–9, 1967.

2. Yerxa, E. The philosophical base of occupational therapy. *Occupational therapy: 2001, papers presented at Special Session of the Representative Assembly,* p. 26–30. Rockville, MD: AOTA, November, 1978.

3. AOTA Council on Standards. Occupational therapy: Its definition and functions. *Am J Occup Ther* 26: 204–205, 1973.

4. Connor, J. *Tradition and change in three generations of Japanese Americans.* Chicago: Nelson-Hall, 1977.

5. Reilly, M. The educational process. *Am J Occup Ther* 23(4): 299–307, 1969.

6. Klavins, R. Work-play behavior: Cultural influences. *Am J Occup Ther* 26(4): 176–179, 1972.

7. Connor, J. Joge kankei: A key concept for an understanding of Japanese American achievement. *Psychiatry* 39: 226–279, 1976.

8. De Vos, G. The cultural context of achievement motivation: A comparative research. In G. De Vos (ed), *Socialization for achievement: Essays on the cultural psychology of the Japanese,* pp. 170–186. Berkeley: Univ of California Press, 1973.

9. Kitano, H. *Japanese Americans: The evolution of a subculture.* Englewood Cliffs, NJ: Prentice-Hall, 1969.

10. Caudill, W., & Weinstein, H. Maternal care and infant behavior in Japan and America. *Psychiatry* 32: 12–43, 1969.

11. Kanemoto, J. *Values of physically disabled Japanese American Nisei Males.* Unpublished master's thesis, University of Southern California, Los Angeles, 1984.

12. Benedict, R. *The chrysanthemum and the sword: Patterns of Japanese culture.* Boston: Houghton-Mifflin, 1946.

Patient Compliance
in Occupational Therapy
Home Health Programs:
Sociocultural Considerations

Lou Robinson, OTR

ABSTRACT. Home health is by definition intermittent treatment. The voluntary participation of the patient and family in working toward goal achievement, especially in the absence of the practitioner, greatly affects the effectiveness of the occupational therapist. Improving that participation requires a thoughtful understanding of the value system of the patient and creative, flexible programming.

The unique effects that the sociocultural experiences of patients have on the treatment process in home health are discussed according to a set of factors that influence his compliance with care. Research findings and a brief case study shall illustrate some of the factors.

A hospital, by virtue of its rigid routines and 24 hour surveillance by staff, often reduces a patient to a level of dependence that almost guarantees his compliance with daily routines. Rosenberg[1] comments on this issue, "The individual who has made the transition from healthy person to patient may find that those around him—both physician and non-physician—expect him to act a certain way; he should want to get better, he should do what he is told by the doctor, and in return, he is exempt from certain obligations, such as his usual work and family duties." These sets of expectations apply to all members of the hospital patient population and therefore they suggest that hospital staff give fewer, if any, considerations to a patient's needs related to his wishes, his ethnicity or his financial status.

Lou Robinson is Coordinator Home Health Programs, Occupational Therapy Department, Irene Walter Johnson Rehabilitation Institute, St. Louis, MO.

This paper appears jointly in *Sociocultural Implications in Treatment Planning in Occupational Therapy* (The Haworth Press, Inc., 1987) and in *Occupational Therapy in Health Care*, Volume 4, Number 1 (Spring 1987).

127

Home health care, on the other hand, decentralizes services, and in so doing eliminates the power of the institution to compel patients to accept and to comply with requests made of them. Yet follow-through with treatment regimens initiated in the hospital or home setting is critical to continued recovery and ultimate independence with daily routines. Occupational therapists find it becomes essential, therefore, on entering the patient's environment, to be alert to those factors that will affect their effectiveness in working there. This paper will discuss some of those factors that affect compliance with occupational therapy home care programs.

FACTORS RELATED TO COMPLIANCE

Medicare regulations[2] impose strict constraints on what a practitioner can do, and how frequently, in order to be reimbursed for delivery of home care services. Daily visits are barely allowed for brief periods of time and require explicit documentation to justify them. However, once a patient is no longer in a hospital, but in his own environment, much of the responsibility for compliance to the treatment regimen is shifted from the practitioner to the patient/family. It is up to the therapist, therefore, to be sure that patients/families understand what is going to happen, and what is expected of them in follow-through for the patient's benefit. However, home care therapists must remember that the power to persuade the patient/family of the importance of participation and follow-through with the treatment plans will be minimized, especially given the lack of daily reinforcement.

Connelly[3] in an article entitled, "Economic and Ethical Issues in Patient Compliance," cited research that defines and explains factors that have influenced compliance in nursing care. Much of the research cited examined compliance by ambulatory patients, rather than patients receiving home care. However, the population studied, patients with chronic illness, constitute a major portion of the home care caseload.[4] The four main factors which were shown to influence follow-through are: (1) poor patient comprehension, (2) social and environmental influences, (3) characteristics of the regimen to be applied, and (4) characteristics of the relationship between the patient and the provider. Because these factors seem relevant to the provision of services by other disciplines, and the conditions studied so frequently treated by home care occupational

therapists, they will be used as a framework for discussing the issue
of patient compliance in home care occupational therapy.

Poor Comprehension

Educated persons such as health professionals sometimes forget
that there is a high illiteracy rate in this country.[5] A definitive study
conducted in 1975 found that 23 million people (21.7%) between
the ages 18–65 could not read. Sixteen percent of that group had not
gone beyond third grade. That same year another study found that
34 million adults (32.2% of pop.) were "minimally proficient" in
reading. That left only 46% of the adult population 18–65 proficient
in reading. Thus some patients may not understand complex
instructions, even if given verbally. Also, there is a tendency to put
more importance in *giving* instructions than verifying that a patient
has received and understood them correctly.

Many patients in home care are seen first when they may be
confused with change of care site, stressed because of uncertainties
related to their condition, or just plain overwhelmed with all that has
happened to them in the recent past. They may find that they have
already forgotten the instructions told to them by various practitioners during their hospital stay. Sometimes, in occupational therapy,
it is discovered in conversations later with a patient that he had had
no intention of following instructions given him by the hospital
practitioners, but appeared to listen out of politeness. The patient
had anticipated that everything would be "okay" once at home, or
that others would be doing everything for him. Only once at home
did he find himself struggling to recall how he had been instructed
to do things independently or to tell others how to help. Therefore,
timing and certainty of understanding are essential in communicating with patients about things they must do in your absence.

Language barriers also present potential problems in communicating instructions. Patients from many ethnic groups still speak
their native languages. Patients who speak English with dialects or
accents are also difficult to understand at times, and they may not
comprehend what a therapist using 'educated' English means. Thus
patients may not fully understand instructions given them by
therapists or feel comfortable in asking questions to clarify. In a
study that looked at ethnicity and language,[6] 80% of those from the
four ethnic groups studied felt that home care services they received
were better when the provider spoke their languages.

Other elements, such as impaired sensory functioning, poor vision, poor cognitive skills, and speech and language deficits can add to communication problems. Patients may be embarrassed to admit their limitations and sometimes cover them up. A thorough and objective assessment of comprehension before initiating instruction allows the therapist to determine what problems may be encountered by the patient in understanding and implementing instructions. Problems can be minimized as teaching of treatment plan activities are matched to patient's level of functioning with comprehension tasks.

Social and Environmental Influences

Many practitioners who go from hospital practice to home care discover that it is very different and difficult to function in home settings where socioeconomic and cultural influences are prominent in the way the patients/families live. For example, there may be problems of basic cleanliness and sanitation, caused both by economic status and life styles, which could threaten patient ability to comply with daily treatment plans. Not uncommonly in working in homes of urban poor one finds roaches and rats in evidence, always threats to health, particularly if treating small infants and children who must be on the floor. Similar difficulties might occur when working with adults in kitchen and bathroom activities.

Patients, like all of us, need to be considered as valued members of the family who contribute to decision making and receive love and respect. When ill, and when former roles are compromised, noncompliance with treatment may occur as a patient's way of exerting control over a situation where he feels he has no control. This may result in a very manipulative patient who causes stress within the family thus sabotaging compliance with overall programming. This is especially true when role reversals occur between patient/parents and adult children, a situation called generational inversion.[7] Most commonly an adult daughter becomes the primary caregiver to her parent, and this can result in resentment, power struggles for control, and may even lead to abuse. Refusal to work with such a caregiver during the therapist's absence is a behavior commonly observed in home care practice. Resistance of this kind can sometimes be reduced when those on the treatment team are united in supporting the caregiver's role while at the same time giving positive feedback to the patient and encouraging his ability to retain control in as many activities as possible.

Another sociocultural situation which affects treatment is the chaos encountered when patients are members of large families. This means that there are several persons who may be present during the treatment session. This situation is frequently compounded by multiple caregivers each with different demands/needs and relationships with the patient. One must devise ways to bring order out of such chaos so that a workable caregiver arrangement can be instituted to insure follow-through with the treatment plan.

At the opposite extreme is the patient who lives alone and has no support system, so relies on the agency exclusively. Follow-through with treatment could be impeded by the patient's preoccupation with finances or getting survival needs met, such as purchasing groceries. In such cases a referral to social services and possibly community agencies that provide friendly visitors and/or telephone reassurance programs could be the most effective intervention strategy initially. Once a patient's basic needs have been addressed she can better concentrate on therapy.

At the same time, the ability of the therapist to influence the treatment process is affected by the way the patient appears to view the importance of the service in relation to other routine activities. Some more affluent patients, for example, may not seem to value the care when they expect that their convenience should be the major criteria for scheduling visits. Personal experience by the author has shown that such patients often state preference for late morning appointments (not early or at nap time after lunch), or to fit around other personal activities such as a visit from the hairdresser. Though these scheduling restrictions can create scheduling conflicts for the therapist, it is worth considering whether compliance with treatment regimens will be lessened by insistence on more convenience by the therapist.

Characteristics of the Regimen

Given the fact that cultural and family influences will affect compliance with and effectiveness of home care programs, therapists must choose treatment activities thoughtfully. Activities that seem excessively complicated (multiple exercise routines), unnatural (doing ADL at the wrong time of day), tedious (working with strange materials or movements), or painful are less likely to be carried out by patient/family. The patient's ethnic origin can surely affect his view of a regimen assigned to him if it violates his cultural values or his response to it is not fully understood by the therapist. For example, understanding the differences in how people of different cultures view pain may guide the therapist in choice and duration of activities that may elicit pain. Rosenberg[8] cites studies that indicate that Italians are sensitive to the immediate pain experience and are happy when relief is obtained. Jewish people view pain as indicative that their bodies are 'falling apart,' so in the face of relief may continue to complain. Irish people, on the other hand, accept pain as a fact of life, and may deny that anything is wrong. With this kind of knowledge, a practitioner may be better able to plan and communicate about activities required in a treatment routine.

Hospitalized patients may comment about an activity being 'silly' or 'childish' during a treatment session in occupational therapy, but may comply with the treatment anyway. With the loss of the power of the institution to enforce compliance, coupled with the constraints placed on treatment by payors, the therapist's selection of functional, performance oriented activities to which patients can relate becomes even more imperative.

Characteristics of the Relationship Between Patient and Provider

Groves et al.[9] identify five characteristics essential for the occupational therapist to be effective in home care. These include independence, flexibility, adaptability, ingenuity and having a breadth of skills and knowledge. Occupational therapists are typically from white, middle-class backgrounds, urban or rural, and possess the inherent values, mores, and expectations of those experiences. When they work in home care, they must serve persons from many ethnic backgrounds and socioeconomic groups. Many practitioners functioning within the safe environment of a hospital are unthreatened by the diverse backgrounds and needs of the patients they see and may ignore cultural sets in planning treatment. They simply proceed with the usual treatment regimes. On the other hand, there is danger, when these same therapist are seeing patients in culturally different home environments, that they will assign lower expections in treatment or will offer activities which are inappropriate or unacceptable to the patient. In either instance the treatment relationship, which was viewed as the most important factor in the Connelly article, is jeopardized.

For example, a White therapist in the Black community might feel that men seen 'hanging out' had no potential for gainful employment, not considering the possibilities of work that required shifts of other flexible schedules that allow them to participate in both activities. Other observations such as the prevalence of television watching by all ages in low income communities, to the exclusion of other recreational activities, might appear that such persons/families lack imagination or initiative. It is important to remember that funds for other recreation may be very limited, as may be recreational facilities/programs in the community. Transportation to recreational programs could be a problem, as it often is to medical appointments. Also, rejecting scrap craft (tissue rolls or egg cartons) as unacceptable by the therapist may not be appropriate if the patient's financial situation does not permit purchase of craft materials. Use of these may not be considered demeaning, especially for patients who have learned to use all the resources in their environments. Each of these situations can offer clues to the negative implications of operating purely from one's own values in planning treatment and relating with patients. It also illustrates the need for therapists to suspend their value judgments and respect the values of their patients.

Understanding the patient's problems and proposed solutions from his perspective is of major importance to the therapist in building a good therapeutic relationship and in facilitating compliance with treatment regimens. Even within the context of the 'sacred' patient-physician relationship, there is now speculation that noncompliance with treatment regimens by some patients may be attributed to the 'cultural distance created by the elevated socioeconomic status of physicians in our culture.'[10] Thus no one on the health care team, and especially in home care, is excused from attending to the importance of sociocultural needs of patients.

Sociocultural factors as they relate to the patient-therapist relationship become apparent when one examines the mini case that follows.

Mrs. F. was a 68 year old Black female who requested replacement of her White therapist after many weeks of treatment. The complaint from the patient/family was that the therapist had been 'condescending.' They emphasized that the fact that the therapist was a Southern, white woman had no bearing on their request. The therapist reported to her supervisor that there had been no indication from the patient/family that they had been dissatisfied with her services. Besides the patient/family's own bias, the thing that may have been offensive to them was the use of the 'cooking pan' for hygiene practice. Although the therapist had not specifically requested to use the pan, the patient had not rejected it for use either. Nonetheless, in many Black families cooking and hygiene activities are kept separate.

It seemed futile to try to alter the patient's cultural set or attempt to salvage a damaged relationship. Instead, a different therapist was assigned so that the therapy process could continue. Better communication between the original therapist and the patient, and more sensitivity to the values relating to personal hygiene habits might have avoided some difficulties. In addition, one must remember that as a guest in the patient's home, the therapist must be conscious of the need to obtain 'permission' from the patient/family before utilizing certain objects in the home. Not only does being courteous assist in avoiding uncomfortable situations for the therapist, but it also gives the patient more of a sense of control in his own environment.

A COMPLIANCE MODEL

Connelly[11] proposes a three step approach for eliciting compliance from patients. These include, (1) establishing a plan and specifying self care behaviors (to be performed/practiced) (2) helping to develop competence in those behaviors and (3) supporting and reinforcing self care. Self care behaviors as described in the Connelly article refer to all those behaviors that must be performed to assure that the treatment regimen is being followed. Methods of implementing such a model in occupational therapy home care programs shall now be addressed.

1. Establishing the Plan and Specifying Self Care Behaviors (to Be Performed/Practices)

The family who has just left the protection of the hospital needs to know that many of their most crucial needs will be met. Knowing generally how much information a patient/family may have about occupational therapy or home care services can give the therapist a framework in which to communicate with patient/family and establish a treatment plan. Studies have shown that knowledge about the availability and particulars of home care services is very limited, but that Whites and Blacks generally have more information than Hispanics.[12]

In assessing the patient's priorities and resources it is important not to overlook the caregiver arrangement and support systems. Although we health care providers would like to think that our services are the most critical in maintaining the patient in the community, research indicates that caregivers view some forms of social services as just as important.[13] In a study of social and economic incentives for family members who were primary caregivers the results showed that when given choices of economic and social supports, including such things as food stamps, money, tax deductions, respite care, recreational programs, medical care, and homemaker services, respondents providing care to the elderly at home preferred medical care and homemaker services overall. When establishing a treatment plan, factors such as these definitely need to be considered, especially if there is only one caregiver responsible for the patient and the household.

2. Helping to Develop Patient Competence

Basic principles of patient education should be used in assisting the patient in becoming independent in carrying out the treatment plan once established. The interrogatives who, what, where, when, and how must be answered. Start by identifying *who* will be taught. Will it be the patient alone, or the patient and a caregiver? If the caregiver is different from the family manager, or changes frequently, then the therapist must develop an effective communication system to insure coordination and cooperation will be achieved.

Where and *what* you treat the patient will depend on the treatment plan. Treatment should ideally occur in the most natural place at the appropriate time of day.

The results of the therapist's assessment should indicate the patient's strengths and weaknesses, and learning style. If a caregiver must be instructed basic principles always apply, such as using clear, concise language appropriate to the situation followed by demonstration. Written instructions, including checklists, drawings, pictures, etc., should always be left in the home for the patient and caregiver to refer to in your absence. After the instructions have been given, verify that they have been received correctly by requesting that the patient and caregiver verbalize and demonstrate their understanding.

One effective way to facilitate compliance is to match the activity with something that is routinely done, such as eating meals, getting up and going to bed, or watching favorite television programs. These activities can serve as cues to do other things, thus minimizing the effort to integrate the treatment plan into the daily routine.

3. Supporting and Reinforcing Successful Self Care

It may be necessary initially for the therapist to take the lead in activities she eventually wants the patient/family to do. For example, if the patient/family have no idea about how a treatment activity could be fitted into their daily routines, then the therapist would devise a program to show them with the understanding that the ultimate responsibility for that task rests with the patient/family and could be gradually assumed. As they progress one should never ignore the opportunity to lavish praise on the patient/family for their efforts, or miss the chance to problem solve with them if progress is not forthcoming.

CONCLUSION

Better awareness and understanding of the many influences that affect a patient's ability and willingness to participate in the treatment process in home care settings helps the occupational therapist to plan and use activities that will 'fit' her patients' cognitive and cultural values. A thorough assessment of family relationships and dynamics, as well as personal values and concerns, appears as important to good treatment planning as obtaining the more traditional information about the patient's physical and psychological status and his adaptive needs in his physical environment. Gearing goals and activities to a patient's value system means one plans and selects treatment activities that not only match his skills but his cultural sets as well. Only then can the therapist feel some assurance that the patient will actively participate in the treatment process. Successful treatment then is more assured.

BIBLIOGRAPHY

1. Rosenberg, ML: Patients—The Experience of Illness. Pa: Saunders Press, 1980
2. Groves, JK; Glasser, C; Kelsey, T: Home Health chapter of ROTE manual. Rockville, Md. AOTA, 1986
3. Connelly, CE: Economic and ethical issues in patient compliance. *Nurs Econ* 2:342–363, 1984
4. Brecher, C; Knickman, J: A reconsideration of long term care policy. Journal of Health Politics, Policy & Law 10:247–261
5. Flesch, R: Why Johnny Still Can't Read. Ny: Harper & Row, 1981
6. Holmes, D; Helmes, J; Teresi, M: Differences among Black, Hispanic, and White people in their knowledge about long term care services. *Health Care Financing Review* 5:51, 1983
7. Kukick, D: Abuse of the elderly. *Inquiry* 2:530–534, 1982
8. Rosenberg, ML: op. cit. page 198
9. Groves et al.: op. cit. page 169
10. Rosenberg, ML: op. cit. page 207
11. Connelly, CE: op. cit. page 346
12. Holmes et al.: op. cit. page 54
13. Horowitz, R; Shindelman, LW: Social and economic incentives for family caregivers. *Health Care Financing Review* 5:25, 1983

RELATED READINGS

Davis, LJ; Kirkland, M (Editors): Role of Occupational Therapy with the Elderly. Rockville, Md: AOTA, 1986

Levine, RE: The cultural aspects of home care delivery. *Amer J Occup Ther* 38:734–738, 1984

Beyond Eating Skills:
Lifestyle Considerations
for Adult Treatment Planning

Laura C. Duncan, OTR/L

ABSTRACT. In eating skills programs, the tendency is to address the presenting physical problems by providing therapy or equipment to enable the patient to bring food to the mouth, chew, and swallow independently. To aid in more comprehensive treatment planning, ten categories of mealtime activities are described. Emphasis is placed on individualization of treatment by considering personal lifestyles and preferences. An interdisciplinary approach is described, as well as the importance of involving families.

Eating is an integral part of one's lifestyle and identity. Lifchez and Winslow put it this way:

> At each stage of development, the setting in which food is prepared or consumed tends to assume an importance of its own. The kitchen may be seen as the center of the home, the source of . . . happy feelings. The soda parlor or fast-food drive-in becomes not merely a place to acquire food, but also a social center, the place to meet and to get to know people. The neighborhood bar is sought not only for drinks but for the solace, support, and contact with a subculture that it offers. Access to a full range of these settings plays a major role in defining a place for oneself in society.[1]

Laura C. Duncan is a staff therapist at Mercy Hospital, Davenport, IA, and a graduate of Eastern Michigan University, 1981.

The author wishes to thank Linda Kamp, OTR/L, FAOTA, for her support.

This article appears jointly in *Sociocultural Implications in Treatment Planning in Occupational Therapy* (The Haworth Press, Inc., 1987) and in *Occupational Therapy in Health Care*, Volume 4, Number 1 (Spring 1987).

REVIEW OF THE LITERATURE

The content of most articles on eating programs falls into one of three categories: oral/motor dysfunction,[2,3,4] environmental considerations,[5,6] and adaptive equipment.[7] Very little has been written about considering the lifestyle of the patient when planning meal-related treatment. Some articles mention a feeding history as a part of the evaluation.[8,9] Stratton states that when assessing feeding skills, patients should be positioned and fed "in the manner that most closely represents the average meal," and that "individual deviations should be noted."[10] Sparling and Rogers recognize the importance of considering behavioral and sociocultural factors when assessing maternal and child behaviors during feeding. They state, "the clinician must . . . formulate an intervention regimen appropriate for and unique to the individual (child)."[11] Lifchez and Winslow give an overview of meal-related concerns of the disabled within a sociocultural context.[1]

LEVELS OF INDEPENDENCE

When working towards independence in eating, therapists must look beyond the mechanics of mastication and deglutition. A patient may be able to feed himself in the hospital dining room, but would he be able to help himself to a beer in the kitchen, or go out for pizza with his friends? Ten levels of independence in eating are defined along with some examples.

1. *Eating:* Chewing and swallowing foods and liquids.

Much of the literature focuses on this level, therefore, this paper will not.

2. *Feeding:* Bringing food and liquid up from the table and inserting into the mouth.

Personal preference and previous habits can influence treatment at this level:

Dean preferred not to use a straw; however, to remove his palmar cuff so he could maneuver the cup each time he wanted a drink was too time consuming. He and the occupational therapist designed and fabricated a device to allow him to lift the cup with his cuff on.

Ted was accustomed to eating rapidly, taking large bites, and gulping drinks. The therapist needed to cut his food into small pieces, instruct him to count to ten between bites, and pour liquids into a glass, one swallow at a time, until Ted was able to monitor his portions without choking.

3. *Hospital dining:* Managing foods and packages served on a hospital tray.

Before beginning therapy at this level, therapists need to consider their approach to certain controversial treatment issues such as: finger feeding, opening packages, cutting meat, and treating during meals or in groups.

Ideally, these questions are answered according to a balance of patient preference, therapeutic goals, and the nature of the group. Generalized decisions should be avoided, as each individual and each group is different.

For example, some feel that skills should not be taught during meals. However, some patients may benefit from instruction at mealtime when the therapy is more meaningful. If several in a group have similar problems, they may be able to receive instruction at the same time, and offer suggestions and encouragement to each other.

If therapy is given during meals, the pleasantness of mealtime should be preserved by avoiding a bombardment of "dos and don'ts." Point out successes frequently and be gentle with suggestions. Proceed at the patient's pace, not expecting to correct everything in one session. Understanding mealtime customs, and the personality and emotional status of each patient can also help.

4. *Family style:* Eating home meals according to previous customs. This includes cleanliness, socialization, and etiquette.

There are numerous ways the hospital atmosphere and dining arrangements differ from family dining. Some of these differences are easily corrected. Therapists can encourage patients to introduce themselves and carry on a conversation. Turning on the TV and drawing out a discussion around the news or a show can create a more home-like atmosphere and can meet other therapeutic goals such as socialization and reality orientation.

On a unit with confused patients in a nursing home, one occupational therapist manipulated the environment. During the noon meal, for example, tablecloths were removed and the curtains were opened, allowing outside light to enter. At supper, on the other hand, the curtains were closed, lamps were turned on, and tablecloths were replaced. Because certain meals are associated with the time of day, it was understandable that with this regimen, there were noticeable improvements in the residents' reality orientation.

A study by Cluff and Campbell showed that, if allowed freedom of selection, patients will choose the same place to sit at every meal.[12] Remembering and allowing for such a simple thing can give a hospitalized person a much needed sense of personal space. Other changes may be more difficult to achieve. Setting out salt and pepper shakers, a loaf of bread, a box of crackers, and a gallon of milk on the table, for example, would require consultation with the dietician, and nursing staff, as well as close attention to all patients on special diets.

The occupational therapist can accommodate individual patients who are ready to practice family dining skills. When another patient was preparing a family style dinner, Dean was invited to the meal. It was discovered that a strap was needed on a serving spoon in order for him to serve himself. He was unable to transfer sticky foods, such as mashed potatoes, from the spoon to the plate, and adaptive methods were also explored for opening jars and bottles.

When examining the eating area in a home, be sure to consider family customs. If members of a family are accustomed to taking their plates to the TV down in the lower level family room, an accessible kitchen on the main level may be meaningless. It is often necessary to consider whether it is more realistic for the patient to learn to function within the family's lifestyle, or for the family to change their mealtime customs. For example, the family described above may wish to move the TV to the kitchen, or they may decide to install a wheelchair lift so the patient can join them in the usual setting. The occupational therapist might present various options, and assist with decisions.

5. *Restaurant skills:* Using transportation, managing architectural barriers, and eating in a restaurant.

People go to a restaurant not just for a meal, but also for the atmosphere, service, and social contact it offers. For the disabled, going out to eat requires self confidence and acceptance as they put their skills to work out in public. They also will meet many attitudinal and environmental challenges. Rusk and Taylor state, "When one of the staff members . . . is dining out . . . and he sees a former patient at another table, he knows that patient has 'made the grade.' "[13]

Bob was unsure whether he and his wife would be able to manage independently after she had a stroke. They had been accustomed to dining out frequently, so the occupational therapist arranged a trip to a restaurant, gave them needed guidance and provided opportunity for them to practice car transfers and other skills as well. Going out in the actual community gave them the confidence they needed. In Bob's own words, "that showed me we could do it."

Transportation and accessibility problems often contribute to isolation and prevent return to previous lifestyles. Many disabled people will stick to a few reliable establishments which they know are accessible and friendly toward them.[1] But it is important that they know how to evaluate accessibility of other facilities in order to save time and prevent disappointment.

6. *Cafeteria skills:* Eating at a cafeteria, fast-food place, or a place with buffet-style service.

Cafeteria dining actually involves more skills than restaurant dining, since fewer services are provided for the customer.

Eugene gets more of his meals at a nearby cafeteria. After receiving his lower extremity prosthesis and some training, his therapy involved going out to a cafeteria for dinner. He was able to practice car transfers, maneuvering curbs, opening heavy doors, walking down a cafeteria line, and carrying a tray of food.

Meal-related activities for Susan included buying refreshments at the movies, and ordering a sandwich and soda from a fast-food place. Both activities called for exposure to the public as well as practicing one-handed techniques and communicating with strangers, all of which were difficult for her. However, the experience helped her to overcome her isolation as she began to realize that her stroke and aphasia need not limit her to the extent that they had.

7. *Snacking:* Preparing and eating between-meal snacks.

Many patients who are not capable of preparing an entire meal may be able to fix themselves a favorite snack, such as popcorn, or get some leftovers out of the refrigerator. This allows some independence without the unnecessary frustration that often occurs when patients are asked to perform tasks which are beyond their capabilities, or are not a part of their lifestyle.

Heidi is a 14 year old who suffered a head injury. Her snack activities included buying a bag of chips and a soda pop and going out for ice cream. Cognitive skills were addressed including: short term memory, money management, decision making, sequencing, and interaction with the public. Independence was encouraged through activities that were fun and congruent with age and lifestyle.

8. *Cold meal preparation:* Preparing a meal for one, without heating foods or liquids.

Fixing a sandwich or a bowl of cereal and orange juice are

valuable skills that should not be overlooked when considering a patient's functional abilities. It is generally wise to begin with simple tasks such as these, and then move on to more complex meal preparation, if appropriate.

9. *Hot meal preparation:* Preparing a meal for one, involving the heating of liquids or food.

Each cooking activity should be tailored to the patient's current capabilities and to the expected role after discharge. This involves some ability to predict the patient's discharge destination, and also some investigation into lifestyle.

Sometimes the patient can enjoy a favorite but complex dish if several patients are involved. When making pizza, Helen brought items to the table and supervised, while Frank and Herb assisted in mixing the dough and chopping foods. These roles were consistent with their abilities and with their expected roles at home.

10. *Family meal preparation:* Planning, shopping and preparing meals for more than one.

Although it may not be possible for some patients to fully return to their previous roles, they may be able to retain some aspects. Beppler suggests that therapists "emphasize the organizational or managerial aspects of homemaking" when working with disabled homemakers.[14]

Marilyn was unable to resume her role as the primary meal preparer, but she was still able to plan meals. Being aphasic, she would select from a file of pictures when making out a grocery list. Her husband would shop, but they shared cooking and clean up.

Dave had been a good cook before his stroke, but was unwilling to do any cooking in therapy. However, he became very unhappy with the hospital food. He was accustomed to a black ethnic diet, but was on a weight reduction diet which often consisted of foods such as fruit and cottage cheese. With the dietician's consent, Dave baked a pan of cornbread in occupational therapy and was given a piece at each meal. This greatly improved his overall attitude and reopened the area of cooking to him.

Food preferences are an extremely important part of one's culture and ethnic background. To incorporate this concern into treatment is to preserve the patient's identity and to promote a sense of well-being. Therapists must take into account both patient and family expectations when planning treatment and remember that it is nearly impossible and probably undesirable to try to change other people's values. When Frank's therapist did not insist that he resume cooking all his meals after his stroke, she was recognizing the family's need to be helpful by bringing his meals, Frank's need for contact with his family, and the benefit of improved nutrition through the family's food assistance. These benefits may outweigh the importance of independence and might even contribute to a more successful rehabilitation in the long run.

INTERDISCIPLINARY APPROACH

Most programs will have greater chances of success and improved quality when related disciplines also are involved. Speech Therapy can provide treatment to improve the function of oral masculature. The physical therapist may assist with postural and mobility concerns. Recreational Therapy may be involved in planning and carrying out activities that involve eating. The social worker may gather invaluable information about lifestyle and environment. It is important that referring physicians understand the following: how each professional can assist in decisions, that the lifestyle of the patient can influence treatment and outcome, and how the mealtime program works. Consistent communication with Dietary and Nursing personnel, as well as with the patient's family, is extremely vital. Any of them may have goals and concerns that are different from the occupational therapy goals. If aware of this, the occupational therapist may be able to accommodate these concerns, thereby enhancing cooperation. Also, as Rogers and Snow put it, it is important to "educate those who are routinely with the residents during meals . . . (since) treatment will have little effect if the resident is prevented from using this skill at mealtime."[15]

FAMILY INVOLVEMENT

The question here is not whether the family should be involved in treatment, but how and when. Some feel that family members should be involved from the start in a therapist-like capacity,[16] but such decisions should be made separately for each patient. Observing the family can offer some clues: are they distracting the patient, interfering with the meal, fostering dependence unnecessarily? Or, are they making mealtime more pleasant, improving the patient's appetite, and reinforcing independence? Of course, the patient's preference should also be taken into consideration.

After the occupational therapist taught Vera compensatory techniques, her husband was able to follow through in giving her the verbal cues she occasionally needed, encouraging her to problem solve, and at the same time, providing much needed family support. Initially, Gary was unable to feed himself, but he improved rapidly, with evaluation and upgrading occurring constantly. He eventually became independent, but it was a struggle, and he often had to be fed parts of his meal during the initial stages. This made it difficult for his family to be involved without interfering. Therefore, it was necessary to work with Gary alone in the beginning.

Most of the literature approaches the subject of family involvement from the angle of "how can the team teach the family?"[16,17] Of equal importance is, "how can the family teach the team?" The family is a storehouse of data about the patient's personality, preferences, lifestyle, interests, abilities, and experiences, all of which may influence dining behaviors. Whether acquired from the social history, through a formal interview, or from informal discussions, such information can save time (therefore cost), and make treatment more meaningful. For this reason, therapists should work closely with the family throughout the entire treatment process.

SUMMARY

For disabled people who have lost or relinquished roles such as gainful employment, or home maintenance, the preparation and consumption of meals constitutes a major portion of their daily activities. Also, as Rusk and Taylor put it, "One of the best criteria of the successful adjustment of a handicapped person to the problems of everyday living is how he gets along at the dinner table."[14] Therefore, dining skills should be a priority in occupational therapy.

Zisserman states that "Therapists must evaluate a patient's family situation just as they evaluate muscle strength . . . or range of motion."[19] If therapists routinely include a lifestyle interview during the initial evaluations, integration of sociocultural factors into the treatment plan will occur naturally.

REFERENCES

1. Lifchez R, Winslow B: *Design for Independent Living: The Environment and Physically Disabled People,* New York: Whitney Library of Design, an imprint of Watson-Guptill Publications, a division of Billboard Publications, Inc., 1979, p 82

2. Logeman J: *Evaluation and Treatment of Swallowing Disorders,* San Diego, CA: College-Hill Press, Inc., 1983

3. Silverman EH, Elfant IL: Dysphagia: An Evaluation and Treatment Program for the Adult. *Am J Occup Ther* 33: 382–392, 1979

4. Winstein CJ: Neurogenic Dysphagia. *Phys Ther* 63: 1992–1997, 1983

5. Occupational Therapy Services: *Back to the Table: A Practical Approach to Long Term Care Dining Programs,* Edina, MN: Saint Croix Therapy, Inc., 1985

6. Kiernat JM: Environment: The Hidden Modality. *Physical and Occupational Therapy in Geriatrics* 2: 3–12, 1983

7. Mills M: A Gooseneck Feeding Device. *Am J Occup Ther* 37: 112, 1983

8. Manthei P: Treatment Programs for Children on Gavage Feedings. *Developmental Disabilities Specialty Section Newsletter* 3 (3): 4, 1980

9. Stratton P, Graci K: Therapeutic Feeding Programs. *Developmental Disabilities Specialty Section Newsletter* 3 (3): 3, 1980

10. Stratton M: Behavioral Assessment Scale of Oral Functions in Feeding. *Am J Occup Ther* 35: 719–721, 1981

11. Sparling JW, Rogers JC: Feeding Assessment: Development of a Biopsychosocial Instrument. *Am J Occup Ther* 5: 3–23, 1985

12. Cluff PJ, Campbell WH: The Social Corridor: An Environmental and Behavioral Evaluation. *The Gerontologist* 15: 516–523, 1975

13. Rusk HA, Taylor EJ, in collaboration with JJ Zimmerman: Living *with a Disability,* Garden City, NY: The Blakiston Company, Inc., 1953, p 22

14. Beppler MC: The Disabled Homemaker: Organizational Activities, Family Participation, and Rehabilitation Success. *Rehabil Lit* 35: 200–206, 1974

15. Rogers JC, Snow T: An Assessment of the Feeding Behaviors of the Institutionalized Elderly. *Am J Occup Ther* 36: 375–380, 1982

16. Godall GE: Family Involved in Patient's Care. *Hospitals, J.A.H.A.* 49: 96–98, 1975

17. Shephard KF, Barsotti LM: Family Focus—Transitional Health Care. *Nursing Outlook* 23: 574–577, 1975

18. Sandler BT: Training in Homemaking Activities. In *Handbook of Physical Medicine and Rehabilitation,* FH Krusen, Editor, with FJ Kottke, PM Elwood, Jr. Philadelphia: W.B. Saunders Co., 1965, p 472

19. Zisserman L: The Modern Family and Rehabilitation of the Handicapped: A Macrosociological View. *Am J Occup Ther* 35: 13–20, 1981

Sexual Consequences of Disability: Activity Analysis and Performance Adaptation

Juli Evans, MS, OTR

Research has shown that occupational therapists, as well as other health professionals, often report feeling inadequately prepared to deal with the sexual concerns of their disabled patients.[1-3] Several therapists wrote in the June 1985 issue of the AOTA Physical Disabilities Special Interest Section Newsletter of the role that SAR seminars (Sexual Attitude Readjustment) and other forms of continuing education can play in increasing one's comfort level and knowledge base for intervention in the sexual consequences of disability.[4] While I agree completely that such continuing education is vital in enabling occupational therapists to play a significant role in issues related to sexual rehabilitation, I would like to emphasize in this piece the skills and knowledge the occupational therapist *already* has which can be brought to bear in the rehabilitation team's efforts to deal with patient's sexual difficulties.

Occupational therapists are adept at analyzing the components and qualities of activities and at finding ways to adapt an activity or the environment in which it is performed to enhance the individual's performance. Cole emphasizes that sexual activities have "kinesiosexual" performance components and social-emotional components.[5] Occupational therapists holistic orientation and academic preparation in biological and behavioral sciences enable them to consider both of these components in analyzing sexual activities. Consider the following two case studies that illustrate activity

Juli Evans is Associate Professor, School of Occupational Therapy and Physical Therapy, University of Puget Sound, Tacoma, WA.

This paper appears jointly in *Sociocultural Implications in Treatment Planning in Occupational Therapy* (The Haworth Press, Inc., 1987) and in *Occupational Therapy in Health Care*, Volume 4, Number 1 (Spring 1987).

analysis and performance adaptation principles applied to problems in sexual performance.

CASE I

Mrs. M had had rheumatoid arthritis for ten years. She was 42 years of age. An exacerbation of symptoms prompted another referral to occupational therapy to ascertain whether additional education regarding joint protection and adaptation and training for performance of self care and household maintenance activities were indicated. The questions in the evaluation interview concerning intimacy enabled Mrs. M to report that previous information on adaptations of positioning and timing for sexual intimacy had been helpful in maintaining her level of sexual activity. A new problem had arisen, however, in that this recent RA exacerbation involved the temporomandibular joint. "My husband is a terrific kisser," Mrs. M confided to her therapist, "but now kissing is painful and without it, well, he has trouble getting my motor started. I can't relax bracing myself for pain."

The therapist undertook a biomechanical analysis of deep passionate kissing to determine what caused the pain, whether pain could be avoided and, if not, what forms of stimulation might be substituted to produce the arousal the couple had previously experienced with this activity.

Temporomandibular joint (TMJ) involvement occurs in more than half of all cases of rheumatoid arthritis.[6] The TMJ is an incongruous joint with a dunce cap shaped fibrous articular disc interposed between the mandibular fossa of the temporal bone and the condyle of the mandible. As the mouth opens fully, the condyles of the mandible rock forward and slide down onto the anterior band of the articular disc while the posterior portion of the ligamentous support of the joint and the posterior joint capsule fold. A synovial joint, the TMJ is enclosed by a fibrous joint capsule. Free nerve endings invest this capsule, a fat pad behind the joint and the blood vessel walls in the synovium.[7] These sensors signal joint pain in response to mechanical and chemical irritants.[8] The fat pad posterior to the joint is also unusually well supplied with Type II lamellated paciniform receptors that are quite sensitive to low levels of movement, pressure change or stresses to the capsule.[9] Kinesiological analysis confirms, then, that any pressure against the mandible when the mouth is open, the mandible depressed and in direct line with the posterior fat pad, is likely to be exquisitely painful when the joint capsule is distended with synovitis. The therapist, using visual aids, explained this situation to Mr. and Mrs. M. She conveyed to them that closed mouth kissing and kissing very gently without pressure on the lower lip might be less painful.

Activity analyses typically include questions regarding the sensory aspects of activities. Examining the sensory aspects of kissing held the key to answering the questions "why is kissing pleasurable and arousing and what might be substituted when kissing becomes painful." The lips and tongue, as well as the hairless portions of the arms, the fingers, the nipples, the neck and the genitals, are richly supplied with encapsulated nerve endings such as Meissner's corpuscles, Pacinian corpuscles, Krause end bulbs and Merkel's discs.[10] These highly evolved receptors are concentrated most densely in the lips, fingertips and genitals. They convey touch and pressure information on rapidly conducting myelinated fibers to the sensory cortex where the areas devoted to receiving somatosensory input from the lips, fingers and genitals are vastly overrepresented. Collaterals of these sensory pathways also participate in reflex arcs which mediate vasocongestion of erectile tissue in the penis, clitoris, and labia.[11] Thus physiological arousal is produced. Learning, memory and emotion associated with kissing add psychic arousal. The therapist suggested to Mr. and Mrs. M that stimulation of the fingertips, neck, nipples and genitals had the physiological potential to produce sexual arousal and that experimentation would likely enable them to find foreplay activities as satisfactory as deep kissing had been. The necessity of open, honest communication during experimentation with alternate ways of pleasuring each other was emphasized.

CASE II

Mr. R was a 54 year old married male, one year post left CVA, who was admitted to the hospital for evaluation of chronic prostatitis. He had no functional use of his right upper extremity but was pain free and ambulatory for short distances with a 4 point cane. A wheelchair was used around the home, a one story ranch style rambler. Mr. R had expressive motor aphasia but his reception was intact and he was adept at gestural and pantomime communication.

His physician referred him for an occupational therapy evaluation to assess his current level of independence and to consider his candidacy for outpatient rehabilitation services. During the initial interview Mrs. R reported that her husband's most troublesome area of dependence was in toileting. Although the patient was able to independently transfer from wheelchair to toilet, he had inadequate postural stability to free the left hand, lift the left hip or bear weight on the right to cleanse himself after a bowel movement. Mrs. R was responsible for wiping her husband and it was clear that this was distasteful to both of them. She stated, "I feel more like his nurse or his mother than his wife." The patient nodded vigorously at this statement and put his arm around his wife, hugging her briefly. Questions about Mr. R's daily activities and leisure habits prompted Mrs. R to relate an incident which she characterized as typical of their problems. Mr. R, apparently not wanting to disturb his wife, had wheeled out to the garage to gather supplies to paint the mailbox. He had attempted to open a can of black paint by wedging it between his thighs and prying the lid with a screw driver. Mrs. R found him trying to clean the sticky black enamel off himself and his wheelchair where it landed when the half open can overturned. "He tries very hard to be as handy as he was before the stroke but he often makes more of a mess," she said. Mr. R pulled his affected arm to him, stroked his index finger making a "shame on me" gesture and shook his head somberly. Mr. and Mrs. R could also laugh and joke about these difficulties but it was clear that their marital relationship was being affected. "He's bored, I guess . . . has lots of energy and often wants to be affectionate but I'm always pooped," was Mrs. R's concluding remark.

A marital relationship is a complex web of interdependencies. Over the years, a couple work out their roles in relationship to each other. Catastrophic illness or trauma alter this delicate balance overnight. It seemed to the therapist that Mrs. R was experiencing role conflict. The balance of her activities with her husband was radically altered from those characteristic of partnership to those of a caretaker. She did not like to relate to Mr. R as a naughty troublesome child but found herself doing so. Her feeling like his nurse, it seemed, could not be readily reconciled with feeling like his lover. The frequency of intimate sexual contact had decreased by half since the stroke. Role conflict occurs when the external demands of a role are not congruent with one's internal expectations of that role.[11] Role strain, another factor contributing to role dysfunction, occurs when an individual is required to perform too many roles such that performance in one or more suffers.[12]

The therapist requested a referral for an outpatient program to concentrate on toileting and showering. The problem with using toilet paper independently was solved by providing an elevated toilet seat without a splash guard. Mr. R could reach through the supporting brackets under the seat to wipe himself. He improved his shower transferring skills and practiced with a personal shower head attaining more independence in this activity also. The therapist discussed with the couple the need to function as much as possible like the partners they had been. This might be accomplished by sharing both what had been Mr. R's household maintenance tasks and what had been Mrs. R's homemaking tasks. The couple identified together how tasks might be shared to decrease Mrs. R's fatigue. Mrs. and Mrs. R experimented with new distributions of chores throughout the length of the outpatient program. Mrs. R expressed that her husband's hygiene independence and his help and companionship helped her to feel much more "loverly" again.

In both these cases the occupational therapist was able to offer specific suggestions for enhancements of sexual functioning based on kinesiological, sensory or role task analysis. Evaluation data which prompted this intervention was obtained in the context of activities of daily living assessments. In both cases patients and their spouses expressed positive feelings toward and results from this occupational therapy intervention.

END NOTES

1. Conine TA, Christie GM, Hammon GK, Smith-Minton M: An assessment of occupational therapists' roles and attitudes toward sexual rehabilitation of the disabled. *Am J Occ Ther* 33:515–519, 1979

2. Conine TA, Christie GM, Hammon GK, Smith-Minton M: Sexual rehabilitation of the handicapped: The roles and attitudes of health professionals. *J. Allied Health* 9:260–267, 1980

3. Evans J: Performance and attitudes of occupational therapists regarding sexual habilitation of pediatric patients. *Am J Occ Ther* 39:664–670, 1985

4. Asrael W. (ed.): Physical Disabilities Special Interest Section Newsletter Vol 8 No 2 1985

5. Cole S and Cole T: How physical disabilities affect sexual health. *Med Aspects Hum Sex* 16:136–151, 1982

6. Berkow R (ed): *The Merck Manual*, 14th edition. Rahway, NJ: Merck and Co. 1982 p 2108

7. Warwick R and Williams PL: *Gray's Anatomy.* Philadelphia: W.B. Saunders 1973 p 801

8. Noback CR and Demarest RJ: *The Human Nervous System.* New York: McGraw-Hill 1981 p 173

9. Op cit, Warwick and Williams, p 801

10. Ibid, p 789–799

11. Masters W and Johnson V: *Human Sexual Response.* Boston: Little, Brown & Co. 1966

12. Barris R, Keilhofner G, Watts JH: *Psychosocial Occupational Therapy.* Laurel, MD: RAMSCO 1983 p 221

PRACTICE WATCH: THINGS TO THINK ABOUT

Wellness:
Past Visions, Future Roles

Karmen M. Brown, MPH, OTR

ABSTRACT. The American health care system has gone through various stages of development over the past decades. The stages range from a physician dominated medical model to the currently emerging Wellness era in which alternative delivery systems are being designed. These changes in the direction of health care are designed to reduce health care costs and also to promote healthier life styles. Wellness, however, is not a new concept. Occupational therapy has espoused and practiced its principles since its inception as a profession over seventy years ago.

The paper looks at the historical development of the health care system and relates the growth of the wellness movement to occupational therapy practice. It suggests that the profession was a forerunner to current wellness activity. Finally, it explores research projects and the creation of occupational therapy positions and curricular alterations to meet the needs of the current wellness movement.

Karmen Brown received her BS degree in Occupational Therapy from Wayne State University and her MPH in Medical Care Administration from the School of Public Health, University of Michigan. She is currently Assistant Professor and Field Work Coordinator at Wayne State University, Detroit, MI.

The author wishes to thank Neal Freeling for his support in the preparation of this paper.

This article appears jointly in *Sociocultural Implications in Treatment Planning in Occupational Therapy* (The Haworth Press, Inc., 1987) and in *Occupational Therapy in Health Care*, Volume 4 Number 1 (Spring 1987).

The American society today is involved in a physical fitness craze.[1] Although the physical aspects are the most publicized and seem to predominate in the form of body building, aerobic exercise, jogging and fast-paced partner sports such as racquetball and tennis; the term fitness incorporates appropriate nutrition, spiritual satisfaction, positive mental attitudes and all aspects of physical and emotional well being. The umbrella term many health-related professionals use to describe society's behavior is called health promotion, disease prevention or most often, the wellness movement.

The wellness movement is not spearheaded by an public or private organization, has no individual as its leader, and has no single definition; however, it is the result of efforts to reduce health care costs and growing public and private awareness, concerns, and activism directed toward preventing physical and mental illness and disease. The goal is to improve the overall quality of life. John Grossman stated in his article "Inside the Wellness Movement," in *Health* magazine, that there is a "refocusing of the health-care system."[2] Simply stated, this refocusing calls for less reliance upon doctors and drugs to treat disease and far greater individual responsibility to prevent the onset of disease.

Dr. Robert B. Howard's article, "Wellness: Obtainable Goal or Impossible Dream," describes wellness in two ways. In his first definition, wellness is viewed in traditional terms, as the "absence of disease or absence of physical and psychological disorders." His second definition reflects the concept of the current movement, "maximum development on one's physical, psychological, intellectual and spiritual potential."[3] One of the most comprehensive listings of wellness elements is offered by Life Balance Company, a health and human resource development company based in Novi, Michigan. Wellness incorporates physical fitness, positive nutritional habits, appropriate rest, individualization, supportive relationships, balance between work and leisure, community involvement, spirtualism and emotional balance.[4]

Although the wellness movement is a current phenomenon, history cites Halbert Dunn, a visionary physician who conceptualized and defined wellness thirty-three years ago in a text entitled "High Level Wellness."[5] Wellness is "an integrated method of functioning which is oriented toward maximizing the potential of which the individual is capable within the environment where he is functioning. It is the direction in progress forward involving body, mind and spirit.'' Note that all of the above definitions of wellness have an underlying theme of preventing poor health outcomes so that one's life can be more satisfying.

However, there are critics of the wellness movement. Dr. Carl Cohen[6] believed that adults are incapable of changing health behaviors and that their poor health habits will continue to exist. He feels that only a few can successfully make changes in their life-styles.

Arehart and Krieger of *Science News*[7] suggest that television influences our behavior continuously because we watch ''beautiful slim people'' as they eat excessive amounts of snack foods and drink alcoholic beverages. This suggest a hidden message: that without changing our behavior, i.e., dietary habits, we should live for today and eat what we want. Yet, we can still look like beautiful people of television. Such a message does not promote behavioral change.

Negative factors notwithstanding, a considerable portion of the American society seems to be entering into the wellness movement in varying degrees. Joseph Califano, past Secretary of the United States Department of Health and Human Services, summarizes the foundation of the movement in his statement, ''If people are to prevent disease and achieve a state of well-being, they must engage in daily maintenance of health promoting behavior and self-responsibility.''[8]

HISTORICAL DEVELOPMENT OF WELLNESS

The wellness movement is a concept that is a part of a continuum of health-care thought, attitude and behavior. Though its beginnings are difficult to trace, the movement may have been spawned from the disease oriented medical model which prevailed during the early part of the 20th century. To oversimplify, the treatment approach at that time was disease oriented as opposed to looking at the total patient, and treatment was strictly under the direction and prescription of the physician. In addition, because of their knowledge, financial prowess and scientific base, physicians maintained an aura and exercised considerable control over the health-care system. Consumers and health professionals alike assumed a subservient posture to physicians which helped reinforce many of their behaviors.

The nineteen forties, fifties and sixties saw medical technology advance and allied health professionals evolve and mature. Health professionals and health technicians, combined with an increasingly educated consumer, began to challenge the physicians' control over medical knowledge. During this period, professionals and consumers also engaged in efforts to enact such legislation as Medicare, Medicaid, regional medical programs, comprehensive health planning, national health insurance and Rehabilitation Acts. These efforts demonstrated a rechanneling of medical thought from a disease focused orientation to an orientation in which the total needs of the patient were considered: social, psychological, medical and rehabilitative. Meanwhile, awareness was also developing among providers, third party payers, emerging health planners and administrators that the so-called health-care system itself needed systematizing. By the late sixties and seventies the term health care was being used by many health planners and providers in place of the term medical care. Health care implied less physician control, more input from other health providers regarding patient treatment and a more comprehensive look at patient needs. Concurrently there was an activist society that was challenging all authority figures including physicians and other providers. This behavior was evidenced by an increasing number of malpractice suits. In addition, the sixties found many people returning to the hinterland in an effort to get away from technology's less positive by-products of air, water and ground pollution, urban overcrowding and strife. Increasing numbers of persons also focused on growing their own food products in an effort to improve their health by purifying their intake.

With the onset of the seventies, it was clear that health-care costs were out of control. In 1983 healthcare costs totaled 10.8% of G.N.P. as compared to 7.6% in 1972.[9] Medicare was blamed frequently as the culprit. However, medical technology was costly; there were excess hospital beds; there was no ceiling on third party reinbursements; the automobile unions were setting the pace by demanding more health-care benefits and the oil embargo put the world in crisis which made inflation soar.

Two very important government reports emerged during the sixties and seventies. Both were sponsored by the United States Surgeon General. The first identified smoking as one of the leading causes of cancer and cardiovascular disease. The second report identified life-styles as a cause of 50% of deaths occurring in 1979.[10] Six health risk factors were cited: excessive smoking, drug abuse, poor nutrition, e.g., eating too much salt, sugar and cholesterol; lack of exercise; speeding and not using seat belts; and failure to have physical checkups for high blood pressure, cancer and diabetes.

More informed consumers, a portion of the industrial community, and certain segments of progressive health providers and third party payers recognized that if people assumed more responsibility for their behavior or life-styles, they could improve their health and the overall quality of their lives. The public's concern was about maintaining health and achieving life satisfaction while industry and third party payers were looking at expenses and attempting to find ways to reduce health insurance premiums and increase productivity.

OCCUPATIONAL THERAPY AND WELLNESS

The Surgeon General's report clearly stated that, if life-styles are to improve, individuals must assume responsibility for their health-risk behaviors. Occupational therapy is one of the few health professions that promotes concepts, modalities and treatment theories that address patients' life-styles and teaches health promoting behaviors. Treatment interventions usually occur after the individual has been affected by illness or injury. The current wellness movement is directed toward the 'unaffected' population in an effort to prevent affliction. However, the very nature of occupational therapists' ability to be "adaptable" allows them to not only foster positive health behaviors with involved populations but to transfer their skills to benefit 'unaffected' populations.

Occupational therapists address problems that affect everyday living, therefore, their methodology has been practical. Because of their practical approach to problems, therapists have often had considerable difficulty demonstrating the value of their skills to third party payers, other health professionals, the public and often to themselves. Activities of daily living, appropriate utilization of leisure time, the therapeutic use of activities, etc., have often seemed too mundane to warrant credence. Yet, a concept labeled wellness has evolved over the years that says people should assess and modify these very aspects of living to avert psychological and physiological disease. Health providers, third party payers, administrators and consumers now recognize the need for a practical healthy approach to life's activities not only to prevent disease but as an effort to help reduce health costs.

From this author's perspective, occupational therapy is an unrecognized forerunner in the wellness movement. Occupational therapy's inception was based on wellness principles as we know them today. Historically, self-responsibility and self-awareness of risk behaviors were discussed by Dr. Adolf Meyer whose philosophy of treatment had a marked impact on the occupational therapy profession. He cited the need for a balanced life of work, play, rest and sleep. He promoted wholesome living as a basis for wholesome thinking, feeling and interest.[11] Susan Tracy, a nurse who could be considered to be one of the first occupational therapists, believed instruction in self-help enhanced patient recovery and she supported Meyer's thoughts that wholesome interests could be substituted for morbid ones and these positive attitudes could be carried over into a person's life-style.[12] Finally, Eleanor Clark Slagle, who was among those who organized the first professional school for occupational therapists,[13] and Dr. William Rush Dunton, Jr., considered the father of the occupational therapy profession, recognized human occupation as a means of promoting health.[14]

FUTURE IMPLICATIONS

Building upon both this heritage and on current health care concepts commonly built into treatment programs, occupational therapy clinicians and educators can further their impact on the health care system by strengthening the scientific base of practice through wellness related research, by creating and filling positions in the 'wellness' market, by marketing the profession as one that promotes and practices wellness concepts and by adapting existing educational programs to clarify and expand on the use of the wellness principles the profession always embodied as it encouraged satisfaction and success in daily living activites.

The door of opportunity is open. Occupational therapists should seize the time. With the advent of the prospective payment system, pressure is felt throughout the health care industry and providers are now required to be more innovative and cost-effective in offering treatment programs. As a result, treatment is shifting away from inpatient and acute care settings to new emphasis on home and work environments as settings for treatment and for disease prevention and health promotion activities.

Research opportunities in occupational therapy and wellness are multiple. The value of having increased understandings of human occupation is now more important than ever. Everyone is examining daily roles and habits to reduce health threats and to live fuller lives. Occupational therapy research could include study of the kinds of daily living activities and methods the profession uses as applied in programs to prevent or reduce stress, smoking, substance abuse and depression, or to identify ways to increase work and life satisfactions. The need for healthful retirement planning is at an all time high. Occupational therapists committed to helping people live independent and satisfying lives could help through research to identify the kinds of activities which best prepare people for this major life stage and role.

Three areas of interest regarding health status where more research is needed are: (1) determining whether active wellness programs in industry help to reduce costs of health and life insurance, (2) determining if absenteeism is reduced and productivity increased if employees make wellness and life-style changes in their daily habits, and (3) determining the best strategies by which people are convinced to make changes to reduce health-risk behaviors. Occupational therapists could well contribute to all three of these areas of concern by engaging in studies of employee lifestyles and in advising on wellness habits. Mungai, an occupational therapist, recently completed research that assessed the health care needs and attitudes of a corporate population. She focused on the balance of work, leisure and self/family care and the presence or absence of health risk factors within subjects' lifestyles. Her findings determined that employees who participated in health and fitness programs had fewer health risks. Mungai was also able to explore a role for occupational therapy in corporate based health promotion programs.[15]

As they move into wellness programs however, occupational therapists will feel a need to assume more assertive postures and to develop skills in marketing and sales as they direct their focus to new environments and to persons with different perspectives from those in traditional health care settings. Those in industry, for example, where costs and profits have always been central to operation, will need help in recognizing how occupational therapists can effect positive changes in their cost picture. Applying the science of ergonomics, i.e., adapting work-site and job function for the health, safety and efficiency of the worker, offers a practical area for occupational therapy intervention in industry. Business tends to turn to engineers for answers to production problems. Occupational therapists automatically fit into such problem solving by examining human function on the job. This arena is open for development and many disciplines are competing for the opportunity to be there.

Another potential for development of wellness related programs exists in community based organizations that are not traditionally known for their interest or roles in health care. Churches, clubs, schools all may be interested in offerings that address health education and prevention. The hotel industry is rapidly expanding usual swimming pool activity and settings, extending services to include exercise rooms and regimens, jogging tracks, suanas, tennis and racquetball courts. An occupational therapist might well consult in the planning of such facilities or design short programs and videotape exercise regimes for use in hotel rooms or in exercise areas.

Community hospitals, rapidly losing traditional revenues because of reimbursement ceilings and reductions in Medicare and Medicaid allowances, are diversifying services and searching for ways to market and bring in fresh revenues. Wellness (health education) programs of all kinds are now almost typical in community hospitals, offering both educational and participative health care activities to individuals and to industries. Occupational therapy departments within these hospitals have excellent potential for assisting in the design and staffing of such programs.

In other words, opportunities for applying traditional occupational therapy concepts in wellness contexts are now abundant and waiting for occupational therapists who are ready to move into the 'Wellness Movement'. But therapists must be competent to engage in such environments. The AOTA Essentials for education of therapists now require the incorporation of wellness information into curriculum content.[16] Without adding courses material related to roles in wellness programs can be logically inserted in existing courses, concepts defined, elaborated. Emerging graduates must be alerted to the potentials of these new roles and given the skills and knowledge needed for them to function effectively in them. A secondary effect of such changed or added emphasis is that staff and students alike may incorporate the positive behaviors of wellness into their own life styles. State and regional professional associations can help already practicing therapists to update their skills in this emerging field.

Occupational therapists, new or experienced, functioning in areas of wellness programming will promote and market the profession's contributions. Thus more groups from increasingly diverse areas in communities will become familiar with occupational therapy, the skills involved and the benefits to those receiving such services.

SUMMARY

Concepts of wellness and well-being are a part of occupational therapy tradition. Because of the current unique climate in health care and in society in general, opportunities for occupational therapists to promote and offer wellness programming are growing. Engagement in such non-traditional practice can not only strengthen the profession, enhance the scientific base of occupational therapy through applied research, and create new and exciting jobs for therapists but also the public will come to recognize and value occupational therapy in new ways.

It is important for any profession to be flexible and to move with society's needs if it is to survive. Interest in 'wellness' is here to stay and the movement is going at a fast pace. If our profession is to maintain itself as a viable service to society, it should step forward and play an active part in the movement by applying its historical concepts about effective daily living and by activating leadership in this area of health concern that touches people of all ages.

REFERENCES

1. Fink, B: Our Appetite for Health Is Stronger. *USA Today*, (Cover story), 1983
2. Grossman, J: Inside the Wellness Movement. *Health*, 13:10–12, 1981
3. Howard, RB: Wellness: Obtainable Goal or Impossible Dream. *Post Graduate Medicine*, 73, No. 1:15–19, 1983
4. Life Balance Co. Brochure. Novi, Michigan, 1981
5. Grossman, J: The Wellness Revolution: Will Your Town Be Next? *Health*, 14:44, 1982
6. Grossman, J: Wellness: Fad or Forever. *Health*, 14:44, 1982
7. Arehart-Freichel J, Krieger L: Televisions Hidden Health Messages. *Science News*, 120, No. 16, 1981
8. Califano, J: Wellness: Whole Body Maintenance. *Current Health*, 7:3–9, 1981
9. Wilson, FA, Neuhauser, D: Paying for Care. *In Health Service In The United States*, Second Edition. Massachusetts: Ballenger, 1985, 1985, p. 122
10. *Healthy People, The Surgeon General's Report On Health Promotion and Disease Prevention-1979*, U.S. Dept. of HEW, Public Health Services, Office of the Assistant Secretary of Health and Surgeon General, DHEW (PHS), Publication 79–55071
11. Hopkins, HL, Smith, HD: An Historical Perspective on Occupational Therapy. In

Williard and Spackman's Occupational Therapy, H. L. Hopkins, H.D. Smith, Editors. Philadelphia: J.B. Lippincott, 6, 1983

12. Ibid.
13. Hopkins, Smith. Pg. 8
14. Ibid.
15. Mungai, A: The occupational Therapists Role in Employee Health Promotion Programs. *Occupational Therapy In Health Care,* 2, no. 3: pg. 68. New York: Haworth Press
16. *Occupational Therapy:* 2001 A.D., American Occupational Therapy Association, pg. 55 and 39, 1979

BOOK REVIEWS

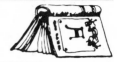

A FUNCTIONAL APPROACH TO GROUP WORK IN OCCU-
PATIONAL THERAPY. Margot C. Howe and Sharan L.
Schwartsberg. *JB Lippincott Company, East Washington Square,
Phildelphia, PA 19105 225 pp.*

Over the past decade, Margot Howe and Sharan Schwartsberg
have been key figures at Tufts University-Boston School of Occupational Therapy in the development of research, teaching and
practice programs in occupational therapy. Following Kurt Lewin's
theoretical work on the study of groups, the authors have now
created both a theoretical and practical book about 'group process'
in occupational therapy. Unlike other texts on the history and theory
of the subject, this book offers creative, yet concise and clear
application of group process principles specific to the field of
occupational therapy.

Opening with a well designed preview of the material that is to
unfold, they present first a review of the history of group work in
occupational therapy to help the reader develop a logical sense of
the process, especially in the context of Lewin's work with groups.
Their 'Functional Model' is briefly defined and discussed. In the
second and major part of the book the authors concentrate on
elaborating the description of the functional group by detailing both
the definition of 'leadership' and then by discussion of the four
stages in group process. These are *design, formation, development
and termination.* As these four stages are detailed, occupational
therapy theoretical constructs are applied to assist the readers'
understanding of the use of this approach to treatment. The book
closes with a chapter on teaching and research. Case studies

165

presented in the research section strongly underscore the basic principles emphasized in the text.

Each chapter throughout the book is first outlined, then opens to its specific content after which references for that material are provided. The use of graphs, tables of information and outlines of stages in each application serve to make the information clear and useful to the reader. The theory of occupational therapy as a basis for design and implementation of groups is emphasized. Step-by-step forms for the therapist to use in working with groups makes this book an excellent text for use with students in occupational therapy educational programs. As the authors state in their final chapter . . . "New therapists are frequently impatient with the pace of development in their groups, not realizing that it is difficult for a group to develop . . . it is through direct experience that the student realizes the power of a group and sees how this power can be used to promote healing or cause trauma and pain . . ."

This text opens the opportunity for the reader to have that direct experience. The text is easy to read and the references excellent. The book can be a useful source to those in practice who employ group interventions whether they be in Psychiatry or in Medicine or Education.

Florence R. Barna, OTR

NEW DIMENSIONS IN WELLNESS: A CONTEXT FOR LIV-ING. Jerry A. Johnson. *Current Practice Series in Occupational Therapy, Vol. 1, No. 4. Slack Incorporated, Thorofare, NJ, 134 Pages, 1986, $14.50.*

Johnson's book represents an attempt to broaden the typically narrow view of health care providers as they engage in the provision of services to persons with chronic illness and/or disability. She has conceptualized this broadened perspective under the rubric of "wellness" or "well-being". She and Schmid define well-being as

a state that transcends the limitations of body, space, time and circumstances and in which one is at peace with one's self and with others. (p. vii)

In this perspective, a person is viewed as having access to wellness even if he or she is terminally ill; one must not be healthy to be well. This point of view is in keeping with the implicit philosophy of occupational therapy, but not with the reality of clinical practice. To enable occupational therapists to reconcile this disparity between professional philosophy and clinical practice, Johnson provides a basic review of the dimensions of wellness as well as basic programmatic information regarding how to establish a wellness perspective in practice.

In her discussion of the dimensions of wellness, the author reviews pertinent literature pertaining to the body, the self, and the environment and culture. Included in this review are topics on nutrition, exercise, sleep and rest, personal identity; these are explained in terms of their bearing on health and wellness.

Johnson also discusses the dynamic relationship of wellness and illness in a thought-provoking section; this section is a clearly presented departure from the medical model perspective of health and illness that characterizes most occupational therapy practice.

A growing number of occupational therapists are realizing that the greatest challenge of the profession in terms of manifesting its philosophy of wellness and substantiating its claims of valuable service to society is the AIDS crisis. Persons with Acquired Immune Deficiency Syndrome manifest chronic illnesses in a way that makes them the ideal recipients and proving ground for occupational therapy as conceptualized by Johnson. For the sake of the profession and persons with AIDS, it is hoped that more and more occupational therapists become involved in the provision of health care services to AIDS patients. For those who do become involved, Johnson's book is an excellent, easily comprehendable explanation of the wellness perspective that needs to characterize occupational therapy services for AIDS patients, given the nature of the syndrome. This book is strongly recommended as a starting point for acquiring that perspective.

Gerald Sharrott, MA, OTR

CONTEMPORARY ISSUES IN CLINICAL EDUCATION. Patricia A. Hickerson Crist. *Current Practice Series in Occupational Therapy, Vol. 1, No. 3., Slack Incorporated, 6900 Grove Road, Thorofare, NJ 08086, 132 pp., $14.50.*

This monograph was developed as a resource for occupational therapists who wish to develop and enrich their roles as fieldwork educators.

It is designed in short sections so that busy clinicians can review concise topics in brief periods of time. Historical perspective's and contemporary concerns and issues related to fieldwork are included in the preface and introduction and provide a framework on which the remainder of the publication is based. The organization into two sections, Part I: Fieldwork as Education and Part II: Fieldwork as Supervision directs the reader's attention to these two very important components of the fieldwork experience and acts as a method to explore these issues in an organized manner.

References are cited during the context and relate to AOTA policies, publications and organization as well as to principles of education, and supervision. The five page bibliography is useful in further identifying related publications. It is good to see these various resources identified in such a comprehensive manner.

Each chapter presents information of value for any clinician interested in the preparation of entry level occupational therapy personnel. Chapter 1, "Development of the Fieldwork Program," should be of particular interest to those who are thinking of developing a program.

The author's high regard for the importance of the role of the Fieldwork Educator and the Fieldwork Process is evident throughout the monograph and provides an added incentive for the reader to either become involved or to improve her skills and the organization of a program that is already in operation.

Doris Heredia

COOKING WITH FRAGILE HANDS. Beverly Bingham, OTR,
Dame Maitre Rotisseur; *Creative Cuisine, Inc., P.O. Box 518,
Naples, Florida, 33939; 384 pages; 1985; $20.00.*

I am sure I was asked to read and review this book because I am
an occupational therapist and arthritic, especially in my hands. For
the first time in many years I am excited about cooking, mostly
because of the approach used by Beverly Bingham in her book
"Cooking with Fragile Hands." Just wish she had been around
when I was twelve and my dear mama was trying to teach me from
Fannie Farmer's "Boston Cooking School Cookbook"! I'm sure I
would have learned more easily and with greater pleasure.

"Cooking with Fragile Hands" is not "just" a cookbook. The
writer, an occupational therapist as well as a master chef, is also
arthritic. She is concerned about strength and mobility, especially in
the hands of the person who is going to function in the kitchen. An
expert in this area of the home, she knows that many if not most of
the tasks will require pushing, pulling, grasping, turning and other
hand and wrist motions which may sometimes be painful and often
fatiguing. She is equally concerned with the physical aspects of the
kitchen: its size; the things in it, and the space between; counters,
drawers and cupboards—their heights and depths; and also special
equipment designed to make tasks easier, safer and less tiring for the
cook.

This is a comfortable book to handle and to read. The spiral
binding allows the pages to lie flat wherever it is opened. The
contents include three major divisions: Recipes (144 of them in 260
pages); Kitchen Photographs and Descriptions (79 pages); then
Hints and Tips (31 pages) followed by a short section devoted to
shopping by mail which can be an energy-saver and finally a
one-page Glossary of Cooking Terms.

You can start anywhere in this book, but I would recommend the
first section of Hints and Tips, "You and Your Kitchen."[1] Here the
writer, using questions followed by discussion, covers many of the
most important aspects of working in the kitchen: your habits and
preferences; then the selection and placement of things—from
stoves and ovens to pans and potholders; and modifying both, your
own awareness of your limitations in strength, range of motion and

[1]page 354.

energy. She warns "remember the kitchen is a place for *you* to cook not the kitchen designer, architect or non-cooking spouse. You make the decisions. Take your time on finding out what is right for you."[2]

Much of what I read in this and in the following section "Bake, Food Prep and Mix Center"[2] made me wish I could afford to put in a new kitchen, a little larger and better organized than my present one. Then I began to analyze my own kitchen's size and shape and before long I was planning what I could do to make it more functional, less fatiguing. I also got a few good marks for things I had already done to lessen the amount of running about, lifting and turning. That's the beauty of this book. You can use it!

And now to the "primary" function of a cookbook, the Recipes. I have always found the reading of recipes to be a tiresome business. It seemed somehow to require a good deal of concentration and rereading to get all the ingredients in the proper order and to be sure of what goes with which and when. Not so in Beverly's book!

Each recipe occupies an entire page or more if necessary. The type is moderately large and there is lots of white paper space between entires. There are two columns under the title (the name of the dish), one for the Ingredients, the other for Method. Both ingredients and method move in parallel down the page according to Step One, Step Two and so on. These steps establish the sequence of actions necessary to "build" the dish from the ingredients, actions such as slice, peel, melt, combine, heat, serve. At the end of each recipe in the left column is a shopping list; in the right the utensils you will need. From Appetizers through Main Dishes and Desserts to Quiches, these receipes are not only clear and easy to follow but reassuring because, in writing them Beverly Bingham has taken into account the difficulty you may have in making them.

If there were anything to add to the clarity and appropriateness of the Recipes it can be found in the section Kitchen Photographs and Descriptions. The pictures become graphic footnotes to what the writer has described in many places in the text. And even here she adds occasional comments adjacent to the photograph, describing the value of the tool or appliance pictured, or possibly the hazard of using it. Her essay on Knives[3] and the list of Safety Factors when

---

[2]page 357.
[3]page 282.

Handling Knives[4] should be in every cookbook, as should be her admonition: "Remember a knife is an extension of your hand."[4] Finally, two of her several comments next to the photograph of a food processor should be quoted since this newest utensil has become such an important ally of the cook.

- A food processor can change your life in the kitchen from a nightmare to a delight.
- Do not buy one unless you have tried to put it together and take it apart.[5]

Having read and reviewed this book I am ready to recommend enthusiastically its use by all cooks.

Elizabeth E. Holdeman

---

[4]Page 283.
[5]page 285.